GET ENERGY!

D1023924

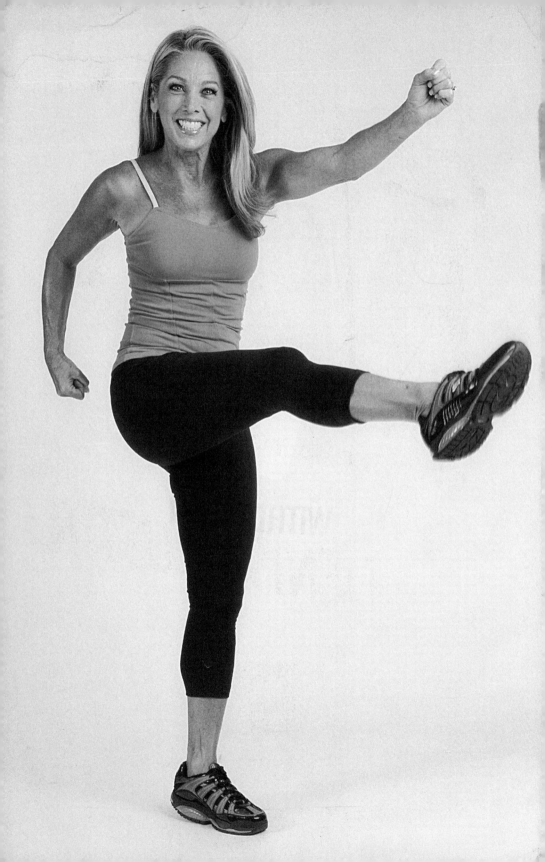

GET ENERGY!

EMPOWER YOUR BODY, LOVE YOUR LIFE

DENISE AUSTIN

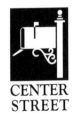

CENTER STREET

New York   Boston   Nashville

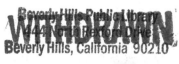

Copyright © 2011 by Denise Austin
All rights reserved. Except as permitted under the U.S. Copyright Act of 1976, no part of this publication may be reproduced, distributed, or transmitted in any form or by any means, or stored in a database or retrieval system, without the prior written permission of the publisher.

Exercise photos by Victor T. Johnson

Center Street
Hachette Book Group
237 Park Avenue
New York, NY 10017
www.centerstreet.com

Center Street is a division of Hachette Book Group, Inc.
The Center Street name and logo are trademarks of Hachette Book Group, Inc.

Printed in the United States of America

First Edition: January 2011

10 9 8 7 6 5 4 3 2 1

Library of Congress Cataloging-in-Publication Data
Austin, Denise.
  Get energy! : empower your body, love your life / Denise Austin.
    p. cm.
Summary: "Fitness guru Denise Austin has more energy than many people half her age, and she shows how simple changes can add up to increased energy throughout the day."—Provided by the publisher.
  ISBN 978-1-59995-247-5
  1. Vitality. 2. Self-care, Health. 3. Physical fitness. 4. Exercise. I. Title.
  RA776.5.A96 2011
  613—dc22

                                                                    2010019410

To Jeff, Kelly, and Katie, who energize me with their love every day!

CONTENTS

ACKNOWLEDGMENTS

I always think of my mom first when it comes to thanking people. She is my hero and is ever-present in my heart and I miss her every day. And thanks to my dad, who was always so proud of me. I owe my "happy energy" to my family and friends because I know how blessed I am to live each day with them all in my life.

And a very special thanks to my husband, Jeff, who has the most incredible integrity and character. His strength, endearing love, and humor support me and our daughters every day. I love you, "Honey Bunny."

To both my girls, Kelly and Katie, who are my Life…I am so proud of both of you.

To my sisters and my brother…I love being with you guys and our families together. That's what it is all about.

A big thanks to Julia Van Tine-Reichardt for helping me with this book, and Nena Madonia…you're the best. I really appreciate you, Jan Miller, for all you've done for me for almost twenty years.

I would also like to thank Christina Boys, my editor at Hachette, and always a special thanks to Harry Helm.

GET
ENERGY!

PART ONE
ENERGY 101

CHAPTER I

Get Ready to Get Energy!

When I began this book, one thing was clear: We're one exhausted country! My mission was just as clear: to help people rediscover the vitality they once enjoyed.

But I needed to learn more about how fatigue affected people, inside and out. I wanted to know how it impacted their physical and emotional well-being, the families who depend on them, their performance at work, their happiness, and their ability to enjoy life.

To find out, I asked those who visited my website. What drained them most? Was it their lifestyles, relationships, jobs, all of the above? The responses poured in. Thousands of e-mails later, I understood the toll that fatigue takes on all people's lives. I also saw that if they made small changes in their routines, and maintained those changes, they could fight back against fatigue—and win!

Maybe you're thinking, *My schedule is crazy. My stress is through the roof. I don't have time to blow my nose, and I fight just to keep my eyes open during the day.* But when you take just a tiny bit of time to care for yourself, you will be repaid with the energy you need to care for others, *and* yourself. In fact, the main topic of this book is *you!*

This is not a diet book—no calorie counting involved—but you will learn what foods give you energy. It's not an exercise book, although it does contain a short workout guaranteed to fire you up. While energy begins with a healthy diet and regular exercise, there's more to energy than that...lots more.

This is a book about empowering your body and loving your life and tapping into the volcano of energy within you. Energy involves not just what you eat and how often you move, but how you think, how you choose to feel, and how well you take care of yourself, body, mind, and spirit. And don't think it's not gonna happen for you...it will!

Believe me, if Heather Brown of Anson, Texas, can do it, then so can you. Let me share part of an e-mail Heather sent me recently:

> I am a devoted wife and mother of three children, ages 12, 9, and 2. Recently—feeling stressed, fatigued, unfit, and unhealthy—I joined your online program. Not to lose weight, but mostly due to the fact that I'd *also* recently quit my caffeine habit.
>
> I'd been drinking five to six cups of coffee a day to "help" me get through my grueling schedule. I rise at 5 AM each morning, drive 40 miles to drop off my kids at school and day care, then get to my job as a first-grade teacher, spend the day with a classroom of energetic six-year-olds, drive 40 miles back home, do housework and have family time (including chauffeuring my son to his sports events), and run a weekly e-mail devotional ministry.
>
> Really, the caffeine didn't help at all! In fact, I always felt sluggish, cranky, overwhelmed, and unmotivated, and had no patience with the kids. I hoped your program would help me find more energy without using caffeine.

It was tough to find time to exercise—I felt I couldn't get up any earlier, and I knew I'd be too tired by the end of the day. So I began to take a duffel bag of workout clothes to school. Every day after I dismissed class, I drew the blinds, popped in one of your DVDs, and worked out right in my classroom!

Very soon, I felt an unbelievable difference in my energy and mood. Today, my crankiness is gone, and my focus and patience are back. I have the energy to take on my schedule and whatever else comes my way! Thanks for making a difference in this busy lady's life!

Heather's life is probably similar to yours—and as a working mom, I can certainly relate! Yet she is now full of energy and joy because she made time to take care of herself.

This book is my version of an energy drink...but the benefits last for life! You'll learn how to live so that you wake up with a smile on your face and go to sleep happy and fulfilled. You'll learn how to think positive, balance work with play, nurture close bonds with family and friends, and pursue meaningful interests and

REVIVE IN 5!

Breathe Deep!

Renewing your energy can be as easy as breathing! I've always said that energy begins with oxygen. Take a deep breath right now...in through your nose...and then slowly exhale through your nose. Repeat a few more times. With each breath, you delivered energy-giving oxygen to every cell in your body, from head to toe. When you breathe correctly, you can melt away stress and relax and unwind—and of course, it all benefits your energy level.

hobbies. Let's not forget pleasure, which does a heart, body, and spirit good!

The secrets to energy are free to all, and they work regardless of your age. At over fifty years young, I feel as great as when I was in my twenties—it's true that you're as young as you feel!

I often say that you are the architect of your own body. If you can make over your body, you can make over your life, and I'm here to show you how and cheer you on. By the time you finish this book, you will have a blueprint and all the tools you need to revitalize your life.

A life brimming with vitality, energy, and radiance is within your reach, and I'm here to help you grab it. Get ready to go from tired out to fired up!

BEYOND ENERGY DRINKS

What *is* energy, anyway? Do you think of it as some mysterious quality that you "use up" during the day and replenish when you sleep? It's far more than that…it's the force of life itself! Let's try some visualization, and I'll show you what I mean.

Scenario 1: You, on a typical morning just before the alarm goes off. You tossed and turned all night, or woke up in the middle of the night, unable to return to sleep. The alarm buzzes, you start awake, and so it begins—frantically getting everyone, including yourself, out the door to school and work, an endless to-do list of errands, household chores, and work pressure. To keep going, you gulp coffee or an energy drink. By the end of the day, you get everything done, but you're jittery and irritable. Now only pure adrenaline will get you through your "night shift" as you fix dinner, do household chores, oversee homework, spend quality time with your kids and spouse—and maybe throw in a load of laundry before you fall, exhausted, into bed. Maybe you crash the moment you hit the pillow—or maybe, unable to sleep, you creep out of bed to watch TV, surf the Internet, or do chores.

This is you on *stress energy*—the kind that allows you to get lots of work done, as quickly as possible, and function under pressure. And when you've burned through it, you're left with an exhausted body and a negative mood.

Now for scenario 2: You're still in bed, having spent the last seven hours and fifty-nine minutes in deep, restorative sleep. When the alarm buzzes, you open your eyes, calmly, and stretch your body into an alert state as you reflect on the upcoming challenges and pleasures of your day. (Yes, I said pleasures—we'll get to that!) You face the same frantic schedule, but you know you will tackle each challenge as it comes, taking breaks to refresh your mind and reinvigorate your body. When stress hits, and it will, your thirty-minute walk or workout will help melt it away and return you to a positive frame of mind. At night, if you're really tired, you'll let some chores or obligations wait, opting to unwind and recharge with your family, a hobby, or a friend.

In the second scenario, you're experiencing what researcher Robert Thayer, PhD, author of *Calm Energy: How People Regulate Mood with Food and Exercise* (2001), has dubbed calm energy. When you have it, you're in a state of focused alertness and are both productive and positive. Calm energy doesn't come in a bottle or can—you generate it yourself, as you'll see in the next section.

ENERGY COMES FROM YOUR BODY, HEAD, AND HEART

Our bodies were designed to generate their own energy, and maintain it at a consistent level. If you're in good health, you should expect to live your whole life in a state of positive energy. Of course, as we all know, life has a way of interfering!

While you can often trace fatigue back to lifestyle, it's important to zero in on which aspect of energy you need more of. Do you feel physically weary or weak? Is your mind in a fog or your concentration shot? Do you feel consistently negative, blue, or unmotivated? In other words, where do you need more energy— your body, your head, or your heart?

Wherever you need it, you can get it. But before you can know for sure which type of energy you need more of (and maybe you need all three!), you need to know what they are.

1. *Physical energy* comes from your body. It's the kind of energy you need to exercise and do everything you do, from laundry to yard work. And all you need to do to create it is pick up your knife and fork! Because food is the raw material of physical energy, it makes sense to choose clean-burning "fuel" such as fruits, veggies, whole grains, lean proteins, and healthy fats. While carbohydrates—especially healthy carbohydrates like fruits, veggies, and whole grains—are the body's primary source of fuel, proteins and fats play a role in our energy levels as well. It's all about a well-balanced diet and good nutrition. Sleep is also important for physical energy.

PEACE POCKET

Savor a Square of Dark Chocolate

To rev up and bliss out, indulge in one square of dark chocolate. Close your eyes and let it melt in your mouth. The dark variety is rich in anandamide, the so-called bliss molecule that is associated with that post-workout euphoria, according to research conducted at the University of California–Irvine. Caffeine and another stimulant called theobromine are also at work.

2. *Emotional/spiritual energy* comes from your heart. It's the energy of enthusiasm, the kind that lends sparkle, purpose, and meaning to life. Your emotional energy is largely about your *attitude*—it makes life the beautiful adventure that it is! It powers our most positive emotions and allows us to feel love, pleasure, and happiness. Spiritual energy comes from feeling that we are connected to God or the spirit of creation, and that our lives have meaning and purpose. When we know why we're here and live our beliefs, we ignite our spiritual energy.

3. *Mental energy* comes from your mind. Ever notice that when you're really absorbed in an activity, you feel more energetic? That's because your mind is fully engaged. Mental energy is the energy of creativity, learning, and problem solving. When you're mentally energetic, you're on top of your game. Another aspect of mental energy is motivation—the drive to do things such as finish a great novel in one sitting, stick to your weight loss program, ace an interview, or study for an exam. By contrast, worry, stress, and negative thinking can fritter away your mental energy, leaving you exhausted and discouraged—and who wants that?

THE THREE WHEELS OF ENERGY

I bet when you were a kid, you had a ton of energy. If you look at your own kids, you'll probably notice how they're always *go go go!* Do you remember having a tricycle? If you have young kids, you may have put one together recently.

We're going to build an energy tricycle to show how the three types of energy work together. Let's start with what makes a tricycle unique—the three wheels. I want you to think of the two

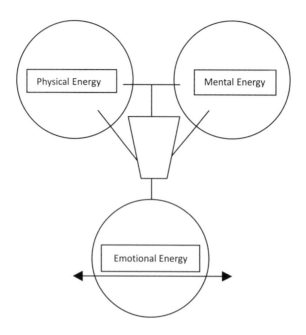

rear wheels as physical energy and mental energy, and the front wheel as emotional energy. Now, it's true that you can technically get places on one wheel—though not many of us can ride a unicycle. And most of us eventually graduate to a bicycle, but you have to prop it up when you're not moving by putting a foot on the ground. Tricycles are great because not only do they get you places, but they're very stable—hard to tip over.

But you won't get anywhere with wheels alone—you need a framework to hold them together and pedals to keep you moving. Your lifestyle is that framework, connecting the different types of energy through diet, exercise, sleep, and stress management. If one of these is missing, it's going to undermine the structure, and either you won't be moving very far very fast, or one of your wheels might fall off!

But let's say you have your three wheels moving in the same direction, and connected by a solid framework. You're eating well (left pedal), exercising regularly (right pedal), managing all the stresses in your life (frame), and getting enough sleep (seat). You don't want to just move forward in a straight line, you want to be able to steer. And for that, you need your left and right handlebars: positive attitude and pleasure, which guide your front middle wheel—your emotional energy. A huge part of my energy comes from these two "handlebars." For me, every day is a gift, and every morning, I can't wait to get out of bed to open it!

Whether positive or negative, your attitude is a mirror into your soul. It shows how you feel about yourself and how you perceive your life. Your attitude also colors your response to life's circumstances. Your life, your job, your happiness, your passion for living—all relate directly to attitude.

Whether you're looking to energize your body, your head, or your heart (or all three), you need both of these handlebars—if you only have one, it's very hard to steer. But having both allows you to go anywhere! Think of people you know who have a glass-half-empty outlook on life. Do they typically show enthusiasm? Do they make changes in their lives that will increase their happiness? Do they move forward? Do they steer easily around obstacles, or do they collide with them?

Of course, stable as it is, sometimes a tricycle does hit a bump or fall over—and you will, too. Many things in life challenge us and are out of our control—our cars break down, we get into squabbles, we are faced with a serious family or personal crisis.

However, *you* get to decide how such challenges will affect you. There is an old Chinese proverb: "A crisis is an opportunity riding the dangerous wind." That is positive thinking right there! When you're riding the dangerous wind, and things are totally out of your hands, there's one thing you can control: your attitude. Make it positive!

Pleasure helps to fuel a positive attitude. Pursuing pleasure means that you look for life's simple, good moments, and then savor them when you find them. It's much easier to maintain your enthusiasm, and energy, when you take the time to enjoy the little things: the smell of summer rain, the utter peace of working in your garden, the pleasure of sitting down to a delicious, home-cooked meal with the people you love.

Pleasure doesn't have to be expensive—in fact, it's often free. But when you team a positive attitude with everyday pleasures, you create a rich, fertile soil in which energy can grow. This book will show you how to cultivate both attributes, and the emotional energy they generate will power up both your body and your mind!

CELEBRATE EVERY DAY!

It's so important to celebrate the little things in life—it's hard to be tired, bored, or unmotivated when you add a little party to every day.

I don't mean you have to throw an actual party, of course. Just work a little celebration into every day. Play Frisbee with your dog or your kids. Plan a date night with your honey. Play hooky from the dinner dishes to meet a friend for tea and talk. Why not? You've earned it!

Life is too short not to celebrate our many reasons for happiness. Too often, we get down on ourselves for "not getting it all done" or for feeling exhausted and wrung out, but what do we do for ourselves that recharges our energy? Remember, "vitamin P"—pleasure—is an essential nutrient, and if we're deficient, our well-being suffers.

Promise yourself that you'll celebrate your achievements on the path to a more energetic life, as well as some of the smaller but just as important day-to-day reasons to be happy. Celebrations don't have to be big and elaborate. Try to take time from your busy life to be happy and to share your happiness with others. Do something fun and unexpected, and the day will be twice as memorable!

GET READY TO GET ENERGY!

I promise you: If you take all that I'm about to teach you and put it into practice in your life, you'll wake up in the morning happy, eager to begin your day. No more midafternoon doldrums...no more falling asleep on the couch at 6 PM...you'll enjoy the company of your family and friends with a smile on your face. In other words, your energy—and your life—will take a dramatic turn for the better! It's not so much that your life will change. What will change is *you*. You'll learn how to care for your body, refresh and revive your mind and spirit. This kind of positive action adds up to energy.

You'll sail through your afternoons, coping calmly with stress and taking life and its challenges as they come. In the evening, you'll bounce rather than plod through your front door. You'll have more energy to do the things you want to do—play with your kids or grandkids, enjoy a hobby, work out. Feelings of negativity will fade, positive thoughts and actions will replace them, and you'll add pleasure to each and every day.

So let's get on with it! In the next chapter, you'll take a simple quiz to determine what part of your life drains away most of your energy. (You may have more than one.) Then we'll move on to my energy "prescriptions."

Each chapter explores a different area of personal power as it relates to energy. In chapter 3, you'll learn about the energizing power of stretching, something you'll find helpful regardless of your more specific energy needs. Chapters 4 through 8 will cover the building blocks of energy—habits and behaviors that are essential to a life of enthusiasm and vitality, as well as attitude, relationships and social support, balance, and pleasure. Be sure to check out my "Great-Day Guidelines" at the end of chapter 5 (pages 91–92)—I follow them every day!

If you're over thirty-five and dealing with roller-coaster hormones, chapter 9, "Power Up at Midlife," can help you ease common symptoms that sap energy, including sleepless nights, moodiness, and so-called crashing fatigue.

In part 3, you'll put what you've learned into practice. To get you started on your new, high-energy life, chapter 10 is a Personal Energy Plan (PEP) worksheet that helps you customize everything you've learned in this book to *your* schedule, habits, and lifestyle, allowing you to generate energy naturally, all day long! You can then use your worksheet to make the two-week PEP in chapter 11 suit your individual needs. My PEP features three daily checklists—one for the morning, one for the afternoon, and one for the evening—that remind you to take those small steps that add up to big energy all day. I've even provided breakfast and snack suggestions, so you can eat for energy throughout the day. You'll team my PEP with the twenty-minute schedule-friendly workout in the last chapter that boosts your energy while it tones your muscles.

Throughout the book, you'll find ideas for quick energy boosts called "Revive in 5," and inspirational "Peace Pockets" that help you slow down, release stress and tension, and take a minute for yourself.

In the end, this book is about joy. Energy is joy in motion. We are all in constant motion, so I say let it be joyful motion!

You deserve to feel joy in your life, and in who you are—and who you are is terrific! This book is also about taking care of you, so that you will have the vitality and resilience to handle all that life demands of you as a wife, mother, sister, friend, colleague, and citizen of the world...the multitalented, multitasking, powerful woman that is the one and only *you*!

You have the potential to reclaim the energy you once had...the energy that powers your passions and makes your life the joyous masterpiece it is meant to be. All it takes is belief in yourself, and belief that you deserve to reach your potential. As a human being, vitality is your birthright, and it's within your grasp—just reach out and claim it!

6 SNEAKY ENERGY DRAINERS

1. **Snoring.** Sleep apnea, a condition caused by soft tissues in your throat that obstruct your airway, can wake you several times during a night. You may be unable to stay in REM sleep, which slows body functions, relaxes muscles, and allows you to enter the lowest state of consciousness. Symptoms include snoring, morning headaches, memory problems, and irritability. Experts suggest sleeping on your side or stomach. If this doesn't help, or if these positions are uncomfortable, talk to your doctor or a sleep specialist about conducting a sleep disorder test.

2. **Undiagnosed allergies.** There's no way you could know without being tested, but allergies definitely cause fatigue. That's because chemicals released by an allergic reaction, such as histamines, can make people feel tired. Allergies can also interfere with breathing, depriving your muscles of oxygen.

3. **A deficiency of vitamin P.** I'm talking about pleasure! When's the last time you had some fun, or engaged in an activity that you love? If most of your time is spent "doing" for others, you may be suffering from "pleasure deficiency"! In chapter 8, I give you all sorts of ways to up your daily dose of vitamin P.

4. **Iron deficiency.** Are you always on a diet? Are you a vegetarian? Do you spend a lot of time in physical activity? If so, you may be deficient in this important mineral—and extreme fatigue is the primary symptom. Vegetarians, dieters, and active women (athletes, for example, or women training for a marathon) are at increased risk for iron deficiency. Other signs that you may be deficient include weakness, loss of concentration, and feeling cold or depressed. If you suspect you might be anemic—particularly if you're prone to heavy periods or are a vegetarian—see your doctor.

5. **Depression.** Energy loss is a common symptom of depression. Other signs include extreme sadness, anxiety, guilt, and poor concentration. If you've been experiencing symptoms and have been unable to sleep soundly for two weeks or more, visit your doctor. Although you may need an antidepressant (only your doctor can say for sure), regular exercise may help boost your mood as well. If you're singing the blues, a brisk walk can do wonders to lift your spirits. Or check out my twenty-minute energy-boosting workout in chapter 12.

6. **Medication.** Many drugs, including blood pressure medication and some birth-control pills, can affect energy, even if drowsiness isn't a listed side effect. If you suspect that a medication is sapping your stamina, check with your doctor about switching drugs or dosages.

CHAPTER 2

What's Zapping Your Energy?

In this book, I want to show you how to become your happiest, most energetic self—to live life with a smile on your face and a bounce in every step! But to figure out how to get there, you have to know where you are right now—which is where this quiz comes in.

Grab a pencil and prepare to discover which parts of your life zap most of your energy—physical, mental, and emotional. Then prepare to take action. Whatever your results, you'll find all the tools you need to zap those energy zappers! For example, if your results suggest that your biggest energy zappers stem from less-than-healthy habits—a poor diet, not enough sleep, no exercise— I'll give you the tools to fix them. Or if you eat well and work out regularly, but waste precious energy on an unsatisfying job or draining relationships, you'll find tools to fix those, too.

In each section, check off the statements that are true for you most of the time. When you're done, follow the directions on how to score and interpret your results. Whether your results surprise you or confirm what you've suspected, turn to the suggested chapter for ways to seal those leaks and take back the vitality that's rightfully yours.

And no matter what your primary energy zapper (or zappers) turns out to be, stretching can help you beat it. I stretch every day—it's part of my personal bag of tricks to keep my energy high—and I want you to reap its benefits, too! So before you turn to the chapter that addresses your specific energy zapper, check out the next chapter, chapter 3, to find out how stretching can help energize your body, mind, and spirit.

SECTION A: *MY LIFESTYLE HABITS*

☐ I skip breakfast most of the time, or have only coffee before noon.

☐ Most of the food I eat is processed—food that comes in a box, bag, package, or drive-through window.

☐ I typically eat only one large meal a day, usually dinner.

☐ I cut back on sleep at night to do housework or meet other personal or job-related obligations.

☐ I rarely or never drink water each day—only when I'm really thirsty.

☐ I need a nap most days, and typically sleep more than twenty minutes.

☐ I sleep more than eight hours a night, but still drag through my day.

☐ I depend on steady infusions of coffee or energy drinks to keep me going.

☐ I often spend all day indoors, and get little fresh air or sunshine.

☐ I work out when I can squeeze it in—usually less than three times a week.

☐ I know I'd feel better if I worked out, but I just can't find the motivation—or the time.

☐ I watch more than two hours of TV a day, or zone out on the Internet for more than two hours a day.

SECTION B: *MY STATE OF MIND*

☐ I wake up anxious in the morning, before my first cup of coffee.

☐ I am constantly stressed—there are not enough hours in the day to get it all done.

☐ At bedtime, my mind races long after I switch off the light.

☐ I tend to have a pessimistic outlook on life—the glass is half empty, rather than half full.

☐ I find it hard to accept the way things are, and often feel helpless and angry.

☐ What other people say or do has the power to ruin my day.

☐ When I feel stressed, I turn to food for comfort.

☐ When I am under intense stress, either at home or at work, I redouble my efforts rather than take a break.

☐ I frequently worry about things I can't control, such as other people's opinion of me.

☐ I get angry or upset when I watch the news.

☐ A family member or close friend has expressed concern about my fatigue and low energy, and suggested that I be evaluated for depression.

☐ When I think of my dreams and aspirations, I'm liable to tell myself, *Why bother?*

SECTION C: *MY RELATIONSHIPS*

☐ I'm so busy catering to other people's needs that I neglect my own.

☐ I am primary caretaker for an aging parent, and I often feel drained and overwhelmed.

☐ As a mother, caring for my children means there's little time left for me.

☐ My relationship with someone close to me—my child, my partner, a member of my immediate family, a close friend—is rocky right now.

☐ When I need someone to talk to or a shoulder to cry on, I feel like my partner or family isn't there for me.

☐ I have a friend, family member, or co-worker who is a constant drain on my energy.

☐ There is someone in my life whom I need to forgive, but I haven't done it yet.

☐ I have few or no friends, and little or no social support.

☐ There's a person in my life who doesn't know I am furious with him or her.

☐ I can't say no to anyone who asks me for help, regardless of how much is on my own plate.

☐ There is a relationship in my life that is bad for me, that needs to end.

SECTION D: *MY JOB*

☐ I've outgrown my job—I'm overlooked and underutilized, and my work offers little creative satisfaction.

☐ My office and desktop are cluttered and disorganized—I can't find anything when I need it.

☐ I dread going to work each day.

☐ My job is so demanding and high-pressure (or boring and low-pressure) that I'm wiped out by the end of the day.

☐ I will go to any lengths to avoid confrontation, and put up with bad behavior from a boss or colleague.

☐ I don't get along with my supervisor or a colleague I must work closely with.

☐ I'm overworked and need to delegate some of my responsibilities, but it makes me anxious to think of giving up control.

☐ My workplace is a hotbed of conflict, gossip, and negativity.

☐ I don't have the resources I need to do my job well, which makes every day a struggle.

☐ My cell phone or pager is always on and so am I—I'm always "at work," even when I'm home.

☐ My job involves endless e-mails and/or lots of phone calls.

☐ I get into at least one altercation with a co-worker a week.

SECTION E: MY PERSONAL TIME AND SENSE OF PURPOSE

☐ It's hard for me to ask for help.

☐ I can't remember the last time I did something just for fun.

☐ I have no hobbies or outside interests, or I let them fall by the wayside a long time ago.

☐ I often fantasize about running away from home to get away from the constant demands.

☐ The thought of enjoying a pleasurable activity—a vacation, a facial and massage at a day spa—makes me feel anxious and guilty.

☐ I've all but forgotten how to have a good time—I don't know where I'd go or what I'd do.

☐ I've always wanted to take a class at the local college, but never get around to enrolling.

☐ All too often, I find myself thinking, *Is this all there is?*

☐ I'm in a rut—no highs or lows. I just go through the motions.

☐ It feels like life is passing me by.

☐ I don't pursue my dreams and goals because I fear I might fail.

☐ I've fallen away from a spiritual practice or religion that, at one time, sustained me.

SCORING RESULTS

Add up all your check marks from each section. The section with the most indicates the area of your life that hogs most of your energy. If you have about the same number of check marks over two or more sections, then you're being zapped in more than one area of your life. Even after reading how to repair your biggest energy drain, you'll want to refer back to your answers to tackle the areas that had the second and third most marks.

SECTION A: *YOUR LIFESTYLE HABITS ARE AN ENERGY ZAPPER*

Don't feel bad—for most women, less-than-healthy habits are by far the most common energy drain. One culprit is no time to eat, or to eat well. White sugar, white flour, and unhealthy fats are low-grade fuel for a busy body and mind. If you skip a healthy breakfast, grab a sugar- and fat-laden fast-food lunch, and pick up more fast food for dinner too often, your energy levels will reflect it. Similarly, if you don't eat enough or eat regularly (maybe to try to lose a few pounds), your muscles and brain are denied the fuel they need, and your energy will fizzle.

Don't deny your body water, either. Your body is 65 percent water, and needs a steady supply of it to function at its peak. Dehydration can drain your energy quickly—and you don't have to be thirsty to be dehydrated.

Another culprit: a sedentary lifestyle. The ironic thing is, the more you sit, the less energy you have. A long commute to work, a desk job, and a night on the couch can leave you too "tired" to move. But regular exercise boosts your circulation and delivers much-needed oxygen to every cell in your body. And don't think you have to sweat buckets, either. I exercise just thirty minutes a day, and that's enough for peak energy.

A lack of good-quality sleep goes hand in hand with an un-healthy diet and no physical activity. Sleep and exercise are espe-cially linked. If you don't move that bod during the day, your mind will race at night. Plus, when you eat well and work out regularly, you blow off the stress that can keep you awake.

If most of your check marks are in section A, turn to chapter 4 for help.

SECTION B: *YOUR STATE OF MIND IS AN ENERGY ZAPPER*

Anxiety. Stress. Anger. Frustration. Sadness. While all these emotions are normal and human, a steady diet of them will quickly sap your vitality.

When you're that mentally drained, it's easy to seek out immediate gratification for comfort. A cupcake, a cigarette, or an eruption of road rage may give you energy in the moment, but a steady diet of any will drain you.

Frequently, negative emotions such as these are rooted in stress. If your mind churns with anxious thoughts the minute you wake up, or obsesses about worries that disturb your rest at night, it's hard to greet the day with much enthusiasm. Further, a glass-half-empty view of life makes it hard to believe that things can ever be different—life will *always* be stress and hardship, and you'll *never* achieve happiness. At that point, it's easy to think, *Why bother?*

Notice those two words above—*always* and *never.* If they pop up frequently in your head, your very *thoughts* can sap your vitality. When you think yourself into a negative mood, it can be hard to find the energy to make positive changes. A negative mood leads to low energy, which leads to feelings of helplessness and hopelessness…it's a vicious circle.

Another way you might lose energy is to try to control things you can't control—another person's opinion of you, the state of the world, a difficult situation at home or at work. To a point, it's good to plug away at a problem. But sometimes it's more appropriate to accept the way things are *in this moment,* however difficult that may be. You may not be able to change a job, a relationship, another person, or the world. But there is *always* one thing you can change: your perception. You can choose not to fight unwinnable battles; you can choose to make the best of the cards life deals out. Acceptance frees up mental energy for you to use in making positive changes in other areas of your life.

If most of your check marks are in section B, turn to chapter 5 for help.

SECTION C: YOUR RELATIONSHIPS ARE AN ENERGY ZAPPER

We're women—relationships are important to us. In fact, they help define us. We have relationships with our children, parents, and partners, with our friends and co-workers, with colleagues in our community associations and church groups. When our relationships hum smoothly along, life is good. When life is rocky, our friends, family members, and others we're close to can help us make it through. But if an important relationship is the *cause* of stress or negativity, it can drain instead of sustain us.

Whether they occur at home or at work, relationship issues come in different "flavors." The biggie is the caregiver syndrome: You're so busy meeting your family's needs, or caring for an aging parent, that you neglect your own needs. Then there are the people who seem to carry a little gray rain cloud wherever they go, and they rain on you! Maybe there's a relationship in your life that's one-sided: You give and they take. Perhaps you're afraid to ask for what you need, whether that's a hand with the housework or a project at work. Sometimes the "relationship problem" is that you have no relationships, which leaves you lonely and disconnected. Regardless of the issue, if you don't address it, it's bound to pop up in another relationship.

People who drain you, or rough patches in an important relationship, are a part of life. When your relationships zap your energy, there are two ways to go: address the problem directly, or end the relationship. Of course, sometimes you simply have to live with it—you have to work with an abusive boss, or live with your mother-in-law. Fortunately, there's much you can do to block the effects of negative people so they don't drag you down.

If most of your check marks are in section C, turn to chapter 6 for help.

SECTION D: *YOUR JOB IS AN ENERGY ZAPPER*

Even if you have followed your passion into your dream job, forces beyond your control can sap your enthusiasm or deplete you physically. They can affect your ability to do your job effectively or enjoy your home life.

Even a great job has its share of less-than-pleasant responsibilities. However, if most of your workload involves tasks you find tedious or uncreative, your energy will dip. Similarly, your energy will nose-dive if you have too little to do, are not utilized to your potential, are overwhelmed by your workload, or aren't given the resources you need to succeed.

High-pressure jobs can be exhilarating—but only if you're suited to them. Nothing drags you down faster than a job that doesn't match your talents and temperament. Being available 24/7 can exhaust you as well. Everyone needs downtime (I know I do!), and when you're tethered to your office via e-mail or pager, you never get a chance to rejuvenate.

Maybe it's the people at work who exhaust you. A nasty supervisor, a co-worker with a negative attitude, or an office driven by gossip or politics can zap your energy, especially if you can't or won't address the issue. Demanding clients or vendors can affect your mood and energy, too.

Maybe it's your office itself that's the problem. A cluttered desktop, a too-warm or too-cold environment, an uncomfortable chair, allergens in the air or carpet, or having to stand or sit for long periods can sap your physical or mental energy.

If you enjoy your job except for one area, you can take positive steps to eliminate, or at least mitigate, the problem. If the issue is simply that you and your job are fundamentally incompatible, you may need to muster the courage to make a change. Either way, you're not powerless.

If most of your check marks are in section D, turn to chapter 7 for help.

SECTION E: *YOUR LACK OF JOY IS AN ENERGY ZAPPER*

I've only recently started to garden—just a few veggies—but I've spent enough time hanging out with girlfriends with green thumbs as they pruned their rosebushes, or weeded their vegetable patches, to know that gardens require constant tending. It wasn't until I watched a friend work fertilizer into the soil that it hit me: Joy is the Miracle-Gro of life.

Fertilizer contains certain nutrients that plants need to grow and thrive, but that are often missing from soil. Fertilizer adds back these nutrients to the soil. (It's like a multivitamin for dirt!) Fertilizer helps all plants, from rosebushes to tomatoes, grow bigger and healthier.

What fertilizer does for plants, joy does for people. Those

moments of intense delight, both great and small, make our lives bigger, more flavorful, *juicer.* Joy is as essential to humans as sun and rainfall are to a patch of roses or a field of corn. Without joy in your life, you may survive, but you won't thrive. Mix a little joy into every day, as you mix fertilizer into soil, and you'll blossom.

Most of us have experienced moments of joy—perhaps when we married or had our children, or as we marveled at the wonder and beauty of nature. Yet too many people waste their lives being constantly stressed out, angry, frustrated, or shut off. If you choose to have more joy in your life, you can. Living joyfully isn't about what you do, or how much you spend. It's about how you live your life. It's about learning not to sweat the small stuff, achieving a balance in your life between work and play, having time with your family and time for yourself, living in the moment, thinking positive, and developing an attitude of gratitude. It's about being open to the pleasures of life. The great thing about joy is that when you consciously look for it, you'll find it everywhere, ripe for the plucking!

If most of your check marks are in section E, turn to chapter 8 for help.

PART TWO
ENERGY PRESCRIPTIONS

CHAPTER 3

Stretch 15 Minutes into
12 Hours of Energy

I have a computer nook in my kitchen. When I'm not on the road, I sit there to surf my website, work on my latest book, answer e-mail, and catch up on the news. While I don't park it all day, after an hour or so my muscles get tight, or my eyes glaze over with fatigue. That's when I jump up to refill my water glass, call one of my sisters, or begin organizing that night's dinner. Each time I take a break, I stretch to get my blood moving again. Presto! Instant recharge.

Remember: Energy begins with oxygen. Stretching enhances blood circulation, which brings fresh oxygen and nutrient-rich blood to your muscles and brain, and loosens tight muscles. Constantly tense muscles tend to cut off their own circulation, which reduces their supply of oxygen, glucose, and other nutrients. Warm, supple muscles utilize oxygen more efficiently than tight ones do.

Stretching also improves flexibility, an essential component of *functional fitness*—the ability to perform the activities of daily life. Functional fitness enables you to bend over to pick something up, zip the back of a dress, or reach for a book on a high shelf. Sure, you can do these activities now—but how easily? Flexibility is a use-it-or-lose-it deal, so if you huff, puff, or wince as you do simple, everyday tasks, you need to use it!

And why not? Stretching is a pocket of peace in an otherwise frantic day. Chronically tight muscles signal your brain that you're under constant stress; ever-relaxed muscles signal that you're okay. Plus, stretching just feels good. During a good stretch, your brain calms, your mood lifts, and your energy generator comes online again. Afterward, you're ready to jump back into the fray of life.

That's why I've devised three new five-minute stretching routines especially for this book. I've paired the morning routine with affirmations, so you can start the day refreshed in body and spirit. Affirmations are a form of positive thinking—the more you say them, the more real they become! My afternoon stretch loosens tight muscles, reboots your posture, and boosts alertness and productivity. The evening before-bed routine helps you wind down from the day and promotes restful sleep.

While each of my routines is different, the guidelines are the same.

- Feel free to do any of these routines, at any time. Start to think of them as a treat you give to yourself. The energy you gain will last longer than the brief burst you'd get from a candy bar.
- Move into each stretch slowly. When you reach your maximum stretch, hold it. Don't jerk or bounce to increase the stretch; you could pull a muscle, and pulled or torn muscles hurt.
- Hold each stretch for about twenty seconds. The longer you hold that stretch, the more your muscles relax.

- Breathe slowly and deeply—in through your nose, out through your mouth. Deep breathing engenders focus and calm, and floods your cells with energizing oxygen.

STOP STALLING, START STRETCHING!

Some women tell me they're so pressed for time, they're lucky to even get in the shower. But I'm talking five minutes, three times a day. Why wouldn't you spend this tiny slice of time on an activity guaranteed to reinvigorate you? Do your morning and afternoon routines, and you won't need a nap when you get home from work! Do your morning and afternoon routines today, and you'll feel great this evening!

The 5-Minute, 5-Move Morning Stretch and Meditation

To sail through the day with energy, you have to prime your mind and body—and there's no better time than the moment you open your eyes. Lately, I've been teaming my morning stretch with affirmations, to awaken my mind along with my muscles. In five minutes, I energize my body and affirm my intention to be my best, most positive and effective self today, come what may.

REVIVE IN 5!

Greet the Day with a Few Deeeep Breaths

You've slept well, but after eight hours of lying nearly motionless, your blood circulation is pretty sluggish. As you come out from under the covers, take a few good deep breaths. It'll help kick your circulatory system back into gear, increasing your cells' intake of oxygen and boosting your alertness.

If you've never tried affirmations, you may feel self-conscious at first. I've found that, more than likely, those who knock them have never tried them. I'm willing to bet that you'll notice a difference in your attitude and your energy level in the first few days.

As you perform each stretch, say the affirmation that corresponds to it—ideally, out loud, in a calm and confident voice. If you prefer, focus on one affirmation throughout the routine, or swap any of my examples for your own—the more personal your affirmations, the better they're likely to work.

Rise-and-Shine Stretch

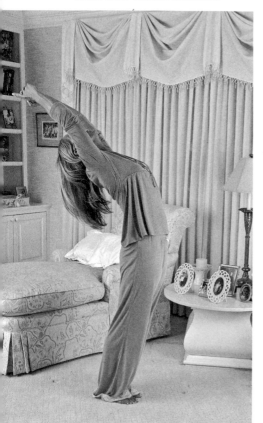

Greet the day with energy! This back extension improves spinal mobility and eases morning stiffness.

Stand tall, feet together. Lift your arms out to your sides, then up toward the ceiling, with your palms together. Look up and slightly arch your back, squeezing your buttocks and looking behind you if you can. Hold for 10 seconds, return to center, shake it out a little, and try again.

I am filled with good energy, and will share it today.

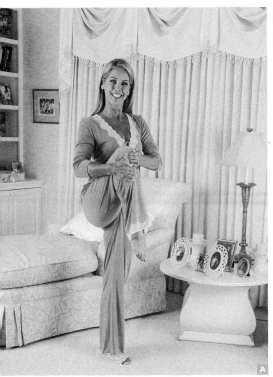 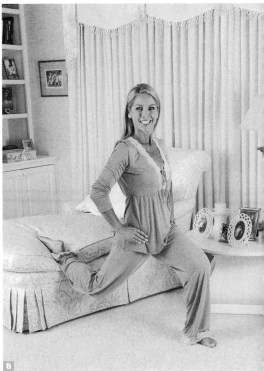

New day, fresh start.

Thigh Stretch

This move stretches both the hamstrings (the backs of your thighs) and the quadriceps (the fronts of your thighs), energizing them for your busy day ahead.

A. Stand up nice and tall, with your arms at your sides. Bend your right knee up, holding your hands below your right knee as shown, and bring it toward your chest. Hold for 15 seconds, then return to center and repeat with your left knee.

B. Bend your right leg behind you, placing the top of your foot on the bed, couch, or chair. Lower yourself by bending your left knee. Feel the stretch in the front of your thigh and hip flexors. Hold for 15 seconds, return to center, and repeat.

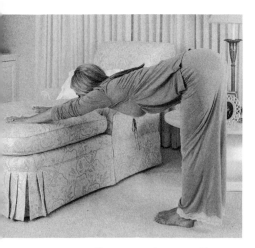

Modified Down Dog

This simple move stretches your whole body and limbers you up for a great day!

Stand facing your bed or chair, several feet away, with your feet aligned under your hips; raise your arms over your head. Bend forward from the waist, reaching your hands out and keeping your arms extended, until your palms are flat on your bed. Keep your back and neck straight as you lift your tailbone up. Hold for 20 to 30 seconds.

I will keep forever fit.

Dynamic Sunrise Stretch

Wake up your lower body—this stretch improves back flexibility and stretches the glutes.

Sit on the edge of the bed, couch, or chair. Bend your right knee so that your right ankle rests on your left thigh. Stretch your arms out to the side, and slowly hinge forward from the hips, keeping your back flat and your tummy tight. You should feel the stretch through your buttocks and low back. Hold for 15 seconds. Switch legs and repeat.

I live healthy and think positive, because I'm worth it.

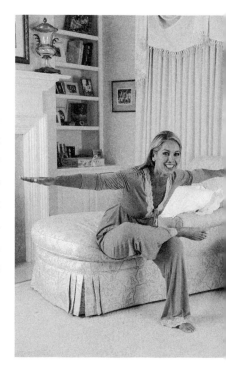

Split Stretch

This stretch stimulates circulation to provide all-day energy as it stretches the waist, back, and legs.

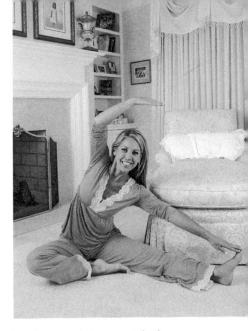

Sit on the floor with your left leg out straight, your right knee bent so the bottom of your right foot rests against your inner left thigh. Slowly bend, reaching your left arm to touch the toes of your left foot as you arch your right arm over your head toward the straight leg. Hold the stretch for 15 seconds. Switch legs and repeat.

It's another great day, another great gift.

Park It!

Here's another great way to add movement to your day: If there's a park within walking distance of your office, take advantage of it during your lunch hour. The walk will boost your circulation, and the change of scenery will jump-start your brain. Take your lunch, too—and invite a colleague or two to join you!

The 5-Minute Afternoon Natural Energy Shot

Sitting all day, either at home or on the job, can drain your energy and enthusiasm. Slumping over your paperwork tightens your muscles and stiffens your joints, while hunching over your computer compresses your lungs, which hampers oxygen from circulating through your body. Result: You feel sapped and sluggish. This prescription for "desk fatigue" helps loosen tight muscles, rev your circulation, and jump-start your brain. And you don't even have to get up from your chair! But you might want to push it back from your desk before you get started.

Oxygen Booster

This energizing stretch really gets oxygen flowing by opening your chest and rib cage, which increases your lung capacity.

A. Sit tall in your chair with your feet flat on the floor. Extend your right arm toward the ceiling, on a diagonal, while you extend your left arm toward the floor on a diagonal. Hold the stretch for 20 seconds, taking deep, cleansing breaths—inhale through your nose, and exhale out your mouth. Switch arms and repeat.

B. Now stretch both arms straight out and up as you look toward the ceiling, leaning your shoulders down and back slightly, to open up your chest. Hold the stretch for 20 seconds.

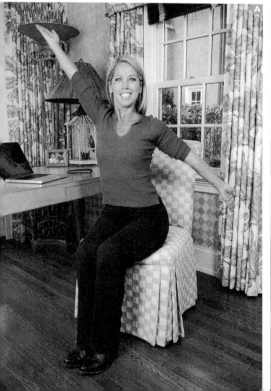 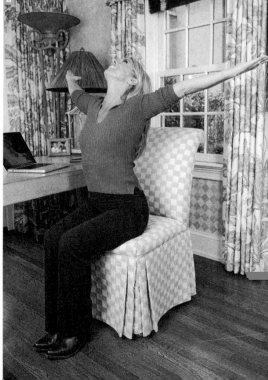

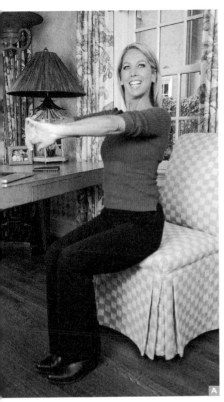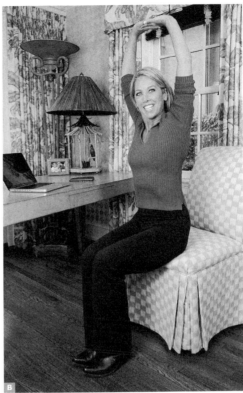

Posture Stretch

Slouching at your desk? This stretch will rev you up as it eases tension in the muscles of your upper body, reduces tightness between the shoulder blades, and helps prevent carpal tunnel syndrome.

A. Sit up straight in your chair and interlace your fingers in front of your chest. Straighten out your arms with your palms facing out. Feel the stretch in your wrists, arms, and the upper part of your back (between the shoulder blades). Hold for 15 seconds.

B. Slowly raise your arms above your head. Think of elongating them as you feel a stretch through your arms and upper sides of your rib cage. Hold for 15 seconds, then repeat.

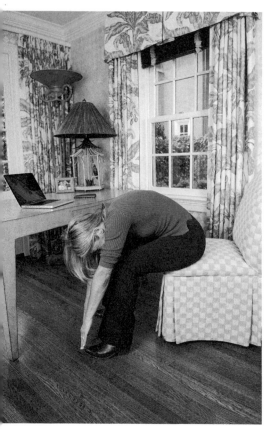

Inversion Forward Bend

This move allows blood to flow to your head, boosting your alertness and mental clarity. It's great for circulation, too!

Sit up nice and tall. Slowly curl forward, beginning with your chin to your chest. Roll all the way down, one vertebra at a time, as you reach your fingertips toward your toes and relax your neck. This takes pressure off your low back, and it's great for circulation. Hold for 15 seconds, then slowly roll back up, again one vertebra at a time. Take your time; your head should come up last.

Chair Spinal Twist

This move opens your shoulders, neck, and hips, as well as stretching your spine.

A. Sit tall in your chair, facing forward, and plant both feet firmly on the floor. Twist your torso left, placing the fingertips of your right hand on the left front corner of the seat and your left forearm on the back of the chair. Hold for 20 seconds. Repeat, twisting right.

B. To challenge yourself and take it up a notch, try this variation: Clasp your hands behind your neck, with your elbows pressed out to the sides. Slowly twist your torso to

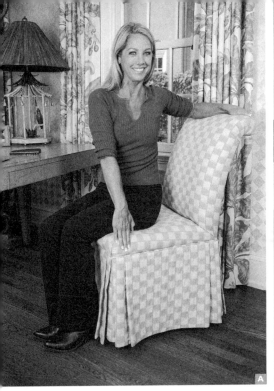 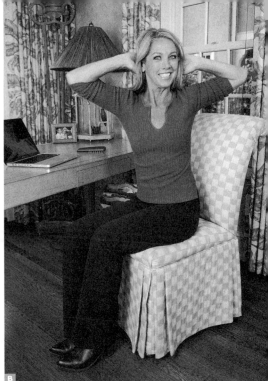

the left, and then to the right. Repeat, alternating sides, for 20 seconds. This will trim and slim your waistline.

Hip Opener

This move revs up your circulation and stretches your hips, lower back, and buttocks.

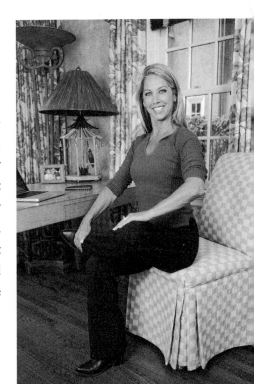

Sit on the edge of your chair. Inhaling deeply through your nose, lift your left knee and rest your left ankle on top of your right thigh, above the knee. Gently press your left knee down with your left hand so that your bent left leg is parallel to the floor. Hold for 30 seconds, then repeat on the other side.

> ## PEACE POCKET
>
> ### Create a Bedtime Ritual
>
> I have a friend who does a few yoga moves by candlelight just before bed—it's a little ritual that primes her body for sleep. Try it for yourself! Other soothing rituals: Draw a warm bath, or dab your temples with lavender essential oil, which research suggests promotes sleep.

The Before-Bed Stretch

This routine will put your body and mind to rest, helping you to sleep soundly through the night so you can wake up rested and fresh for the morning.

Foot and Leg Rejuvenator

This stretch relaxes tired leg muscles and increases the blood flow to your legs.

A. Sit at the edge of your bed, couch, or chair. Pull your right knee up toward your chest as you place both hands under your foot. Give your foot a mini massage.

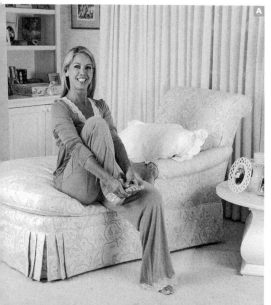 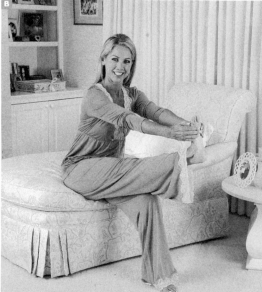

B. Holding your right foot with the fingers of both hands, slowly and gently extend and straighten the leg. Flex your foot and stretch your leg. This stretches your calf, Achilles tendon, and foot. Hold for 15 seconds, relax, and repeat with your left leg.

Low Lunge

This stretch loosens and lengthens your hip flexors, which become short and tight when you sit all day.

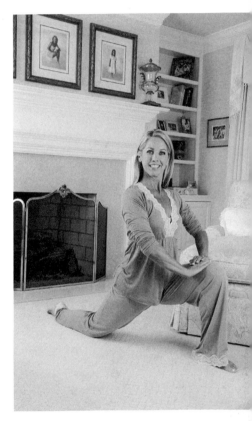

Stand with your feet aligned under your hips and your arms at your sides. With your right foot, take a large step backward. Bend your left knee so that it forms a ninety-degree angle to the floor as you lower your right knee to the floor, with the top of your foot also resting on the floor. Place both of your hands just above your bent left knee, with your left hand on top of your right. Hold for 30 seconds. Switch sides and repeat.

Hip Opener

One of my favorite stretches, this stretches your back and legs and opens your hips.

A. Sit cross-legged on the floor by bending your right leg and gently placing your right ankle on top of your left thigh. Position your right hand on your right knee and left hand

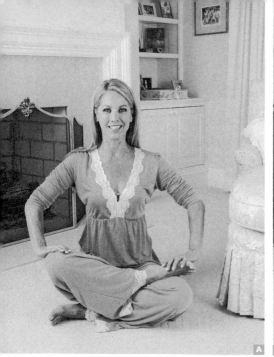 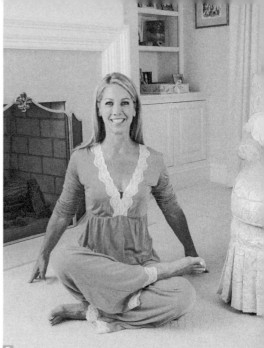

A B

on your right foot. Gently press down to feel the stretch in your buttocks and hips, holding for 15 seconds.

B. Place your hands behind you to open up your chest and feel the stretch through your buttocks and hips. Hold for 15 seconds. Repeat on the other side.

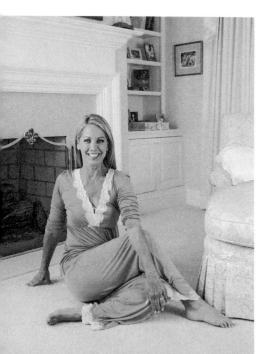

Gentle Spinal Twist

Your spine and the backs of your legs will feel loose and relaxed after this easy stretch!

Sit up nice and tall on the floor. Bend your left knee and bring the sole of your foot under your right thigh. Bend your right knee up and over your left knee and place your right foot on the floor on the opposite side of your left knee. Place your right hand on the floor behind you to support your back. Rest your left arm on the outside of your right knee to help anchor your torso. Turn and twist your upper body to the right, using your left arm to help you lift your spine. Try to keep your shoulders down and your abs tight as you twist your spine farther to the right. Lengthen your spine and hold the pose for 20 seconds, taking deep cleansing breaths—in and out through your nose. Relax and repeat on the opposite side.

Leg and Back Relaxer

This move will stretch your legs and ease any stiffness, especially if you've been on your feet all day.

A. Lie on your back on your bed, with your arms at your sides. Raise your legs and point your toes toward the ceiling as you rotate your ankles, circling clockwise for 10 seconds and then counterclockwise for 10 seconds.

B. Bend your left knee and place your left foot on the bed as you wrap your hands around your right leg just above your ankle, stretching your extended right leg. Hold for 20 seconds, then switch legs.

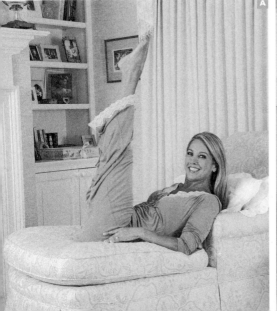
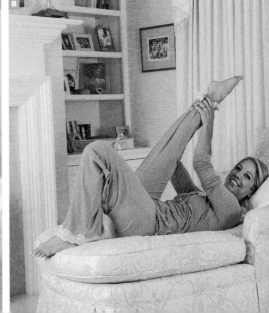

C. Lower both knees to your chest and wrap your arms around them, feeling the stretch in your spine. Hold for 20 seconds.

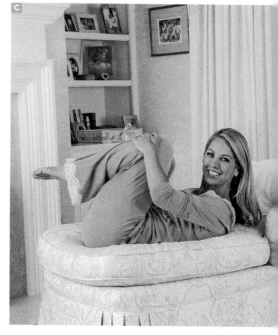

Now you're ready for a restful night's sleep. While lying on your back, relax your arms and legs. Your palms should face the ceiling. Keep your eyes closed, and relax your facial muscles. Feel the stillness in your body—this is your peaceful time.

Breathe slowly and deeply, inhaling and exhaling through your nose. If your mind wanders to the worries of the day, refocus on the rhythm of your breath until you are completely relaxed. Sweet dreams!

CHAPTER 4

The Building Blocks of All-Day Energy

Imagine waking up in the morning looking forward to the day ahead, moving through your day feeling positive and productive, and ending the day with energy in reserve, so you can play with the kids, enjoy a hobby, or get in that thirty-minute workout. Well, stop imagining—you're about to take action and make it happen!

As a working mom, I have the same can't-say-no commitments to family, friends, kids, and work as you do. But I've learned to live in a way that replenishes rather than depletes my energy, despite the many demands my life heaps on me. Yes, I learned, and you can, too. The first "lesson"—that first step on the path to a more vital, high-energy life—is to master the basics.

These simple but powerful energy prescriptions for reviving your body, mind, and spirit are the foundation of all-day energy on which I've built a life filled with positivity and joy—and they work for virtually everyone. While some of them are simple, that doesn't mean they're easy; it will take determination and practice to integrate them into your life. But keep trying. Sooner than you think, they'll become second nature. You're likely to feel more energetic and alive than you have in years. Read through this "express program," commit to it, then invite a tired friend to change along with you!

STRAIGHTEN UP!

There is a proverb I love: "Life is in the breath—he who half breathes half lives." How true! Oxygen is the key to energy. How do you get that oxygen to flow? Well, one way is to exercise. Another way: good posture—sit and stand up straight. It's as simple as that, really!

Here's why: When you slouch or slump, you reduce the space in your chest cavity, which means that you take shallow breaths instead of full, deep, oxygen-rich breaths. Your cells—which need lots of oxygen to function at their peak—are forced to operate on an oxygen deficit, and you poop out. Other consequences of poor posture include an achy back, headache, and neck or shoulder pain, all of which further sap your energy.

When you sit and stand tall, you open that chest cavity right up. This can increase the amount of oxygen your lungs take in by as much as 30 percent. The better your posture, the more oxygen—and energy!—is available to your muscles and brain. Your lung capacity increases. Your energy level skyrockets. You're more alert and feel more positive.

Recent research suggests that good posture can affect how we think about ourselves, too. In a study at Ohio State University, seventy-one students were told to sit up straight and push out their chest, or to slouch. They were then asked about positive or negative traits they'd show as a hypothetical future employee.

"Their confident, upright posture gave them more confidence in their own thoughts, whether they were positive or negative," says lead researcher Richard Petty. "People assume their confidence is coming from their own thoughts. They don't realize their posture is affecting how much they believe in what they're thinking."

Here are two tricks some singers use to really breathe deep through posture. The first is to stand with your heels, shoulders, and as much of your back as possible against a wall, then step away. The second is to bring your fingertips together in

REVIVE IN 5!

Do a Posture Scan

Actually, it takes just seconds to check your posture and keep energy-ebbing aches and pains at bay. Check yourself from head to toe every so often—head, neck, shoulders, spine, tummy, knees.

- **Standing up?** Tuck in those abs as you keep your head high, chin forward, shoulders back, and chest out.
- **Sitting at home or work?** Use a chair with firm lower-back support. Adjust the chair so the desk or tabletop is elbow-high, and keep your knees a little higher than your hips. You can also use a footrest to keep pressure off the backs of your legs if you can't adjust the chair to raise your knees. Be sure to get up and stretch frequently—every hour if you sit for long periods.
- **In bed?** Sleep on your side with your knees bent. Support your head with a pillow so it is level with your spine. If you sleep on your back, use a small pillow under your neck. (And if you sleep on your belly, try the positions above. They're better for your posture, and you'll wake up to fewer creases and furrows, too!)
- **In the car?** Keep your seat at a ninety-degree angle and your knees level with your hips. For extra support, you might tuck a small pillow behind your lower back. Finally, tilt your rearview mirror up a bit—you'll automatically sit up straighter to see out the back window.

front of you as if you're hugging a giant beach ball. Raise your hands together over your head, then separate and bring them down to your sides. Both these tricks will end with your back straight, your shoulders back, your tummy tucked, and your chest out.

While it takes attention and patience to improve your posture, you reap so many benefits: more energy, less stress, and less fatigue.

PUMP UP YOUR DIET—EAT FOR ENERGY!

If you're low in energy, poor nutrition may be the problem. The good news is that a well-balanced diet can dramatically improve energy levels. Changing the fuel you give your body can be especially helpful if your current diet is built around take-out and junk food. Here's a cheat sheet on what to eat, along with recommendations from major health associations, including the American Heart Association.

- **Carbohydrates** are your body's main source of energy. There are two basic types. *Complex carbohydrates*—which I like to call good carbohydrates—are good for your body, fill your tummy, and boost your energy. Foods high in complex carbohydrates include beans, whole grains, and veggies. *Simple carbohydrates* are foods like candy bars, cookies, and soft drinks that contain a lot of empty calories in the form of sugar (along with high-fructose corn syrup). Unlike complex carbohydrates, simple carbs do little to nourish your body, and while they provide a quick surge of energy, an equally quick crash will follow. So don't get on that roller coaster!

  What the experts say: From 45 to 65 percent of your daily calories should come from carbohydrates. Emphasize complex carbs, which contain healthy, satisfying fiber, and limit simple carbohydrates.

Best sources: Fruits, veggies, high-fiber cereals, beans.

- **Protein** is your body's main building material; it assists in growth, transports vitamins, supports hormones, and helps us hold on to lean muscle. Protein sources include both plant and animal products. Legumes, poultry, seafood, meat, eggs, and dairy products are good sources of protein. While you don't want to eat too much protein—especially fatty red meat and whole dairy—it's important to get enough. If you are a vegetarian, be sure to get enough protein from plant sources—beans, nuts, and soy are all good.

  What the experts say: Protein should account for 10 to 35 percent of your total daily calories. Choose plant sources of protein, such as beans, lentils, and soy, as well as lean meats, skinless poultry, and fish.

  Best sources: Poultry, fish, shellfish, egg whites, soy, low-fat milk and yogurt, low-fat cheese, lean red meats, lean pork.

- **Fats** aren't evil—in fact, they help your body absorb vitamins and help keep your immune system working. They are a concentrated source of energy, though—a nice way to say they contain a lot of calories! So eat small portions of mostly healthy unsaturated and polyunsaturated fats, including nuts; olive, canola, and fish oils; avocados; and flaxseed. The fats to limit are saturated fats, which are found in animal foods like butter, cheese, whole milk, and bacon. You should also steer clear of trans fats—vegetable fats pumped up with hydrogen— which are found in commercial baked and fried foods like doughnuts and french fries. Both saturated and trans fats are bad for your heart and blood cholesterol levels. You don't have to give up bacon, though—just strike a balance between good fats and the less healthy ones.

What the experts say: From 20 to 35 percent of your total daily calories should come from fats, mostly the healthy ones. Keep your daily intake of saturated fat to no more than 7 percent of your total calories, and trans fat to no more than 1 percent of your total calories.

Best sources: Avocados, nuts, certain vegetable oils (olive, canola, safflower).

- **Fiber** (my grandma called it "roughage") is the part of plant foods that your body can't digest and absorb. There are two types. *Insoluble fiber,* available in whole grains and veggies, is the type that helps keep you regular. *Soluble fiber,* found in oatmeal, dried beans, and some fruits like apples and oranges, can help keep your blood sugar and cholesterol levels in check.

  What the experts say: Women should eat from twenty-one to twenty-five grams of fiber a day; men, thirty to thirty-eight grams a day.

  Best sources: Fruits, veggies, whole grains (oatmeal, brown rice, barley).

Rev Up with Breakfast

When I wake up, I'm *starving.* I can't wait for breakfast. Sometimes I enjoy egg whites and salsa with whole-grain toast, or oatmeal with fresh berries and low-fat yogurt, or a slice of whole-grain toast with natural peanut butter. (And I savor my one cup of coffee!)

So I enjoy breakfast, and make time for it. I make sure my daughters eat it, too. But all too many people don't—and short-circuit their energy stores. When you pass up breakfast, you deny your body—particularly your brain—the chance to refuel after a long night of repair and restoration. If you don't feed your brain, literally, in the morning, your alertness and concentration can suffer.

Not eating breakfast can also impede weight loss. Sooner or later, your hunger will catch up with you, and you're likely to scarf anything that isn't nailed down, like chocolate kisses from a co-worker's candy jar or a doughnut from the office vending machines. Further, prolonged fasting—which is what skipping breakfast is—can increase your body's response to insulin, which in turn increases the storage of body fat. In fact, research suggests that skipping breakfast can raise the risk of obesity.

On the other hand, studies have found that people who eat breakfast regularly enjoy more energy and a better mood throughout the day. Breakfast gives your brain and muscles the fuel they need for the day ahead, revs your metabolism, and keeps your hunger in check, so you're less likely to overeat at lunch or dinner.

Make sure your breakfast contains plenty of fiber and nutrients via healthy complex carbohydrates, which are energy foods! A serving of high-fiber, low-sugar cereal with berries and skim milk has the perfect balance of protein and carbohydrate that will help keep you energy-high throughout the morning. The bread and cereal you choose should contain three grams of fiber per serving, so check the nutrition labels.

A healthy breakfast, and a healthy diet in general, also contains small portions of good fats—think nuts, organic almond or natural peanut butter, avocados, olive oil, flaxseed oil, or canola oil—and lean protein, such as egg whites, skim milk, and low-fat cheese. If you don't like traditional breakfast foods, think outside the cereal box or egg carton. If you want a slice of last night's leftover cheese pizza, more power to you!

If you don't eat breakfast now, start small. Even a little something—a hard-boiled egg, a fruit smoothie with yogurt—will refuel your brain and fire up your metabolism.

Energize Your Diet with Carbs

Yes, you heard right. They've been the bad guy for too long, and it's high time we rediscovered their benefits. But first, let's dismiss a big misconception about carbs: that they make you sluggish.

We've all indulged in a huge plate of pasta and suffered the consequences: that state of heavy-lidded lethargy laughingly referred to as a "carb coma." Of course, it's no laughing matter if you have to struggle to stay vertical after a huge, carb-rich meal when you have a meeting to attend, a house to clean, a workout to do, or errands to run.

But here's the good news: Just as you can eat yourself into a droopy, draggy daze, you can use the good carbs to achieve a state of calm alertness and steady energy throughout the day.

I believe in eating good carbohydrates like fruits, vegetables, and yes, even potatoes. I never take those out of my diet. Carbs are your body's preferred source of fuel, which makes them the best foods to boost your energy levels and brighten your mood. And let's not forget fiber—it slows digestion, and thus provides you a more steady supply of energy throughout the day. Team complex carbs with moderate portions of lean proteins and healthy fats—a turkey sandwich on whole-grain bread, for example, or stir-fried veggies with chicken—and you're ready for takeoff!

I recommend that, more often than not, you select the whole grains themselves (with no or a very small amount of added fat) rather than *products* made with whole grains (breads, cookies, muffins, rolls, crackers, and so on). When you opt for oatmeal over an oat bran muffin or oatmeal cookie, or brown rice over a whole-grain bagel, you're nourishing your body with serious energy food, without added sugar, white flour, additives, or preservatives. What's more, your body absorbs whole grains more slowly, which helps keep blood sugar and energy levels stable.

Now, there can be too much of a good thing, so enjoy carbs in reasonable portions—about 150 grams a day, primarily complex carbs. That's roughly seven servings of fruit and veggies, and three to four servings of bread, pasta, and cereal (preferably made with whole grains). But if you get in a serving of fruit and veggies at every meal and snack, and "spend" your carbs on meals rather than snacks, you've got it. It's that simple!

What Makes a Whole Grain "Whole"?

All grains start out as whole grains. That is, they contain the three main parts of any grain: the bran, the endosperm, and the

Top 10 Rev-You-Up Carbs

Natural, nutritious, energizing, and delicious, complex carbs are easy to spot: They're the foods that come "wrapped" in their natural "packaging"—such as grain hulls or fruit or vegetable peels—rather than boxes or bags. Boost the nutrition in your diet—and your energy—with these rev-you-up foods.

1. Black beans (any kind of beans, actually!).
2. Brown rice.
3. Greens. Pick your favorites—spinach, collard or mustard greens, kale, Swiss chard, and so on.
4. Crayon-colored fruits—berries, oranges, tomatoes.
5. Brilliant-colored veggies—eggplant, red/yellow/orange bell peppers, sweet potatoes.
6. Oatmeal.
7. Popcorn (air-popped, with a few spritzes of liquid butter).
8. Potatoes—small- to medium-size, and "naked" rather than "loaded." (Of course I love my Idaho potatoes!)
9. Quinoa.
10. Whole wheat.

germ. The outer bran is packed with fiber, B vitamins, minerals, and health-promoting plant substances (phytochemicals). The bulk of the grain, the endosperm, is full of complex carbohydrates and protein. The germ is rich in B vitamins, antioxidants such as vitamin E, trace minerals, and healthy fats.

Grains that are turned into white flour ("refined") are stripped of the germ and bran, leaving only the endosperm. Unfortunately, removing the germ and bran reduces a grain's nutrient content by 25 to 90 percent. That's why it's smart to eat mostly whole grains— you get the full benefit of their nutrients.

Drink Up!

At home or on the road, I'm never without a glass or a bottle of water (although I try to stick to glasses—better for the environment). Drinking sixty-four ounces of water a day is one of the keys to my boundless energy, and I guarantee you, water is one of the easiest, cheapest fixes for fatigue. Your body is two-thirds water, after all, so it depends on this precious fluid to function at its peak—and to keep you alert and energized.

Water truly is the essence of life, and of energy. Even mild dehydration can reduce blood flow to your organs, which slows down your brain and saps your energy. A recent study from Tufts University found that mild dehydration—a loss of just 1 to 2 percent of body weight as water—was enough to impair thinking. In another study, of athletes, researchers found that 92 percent felt fatigued after they limited fluids and foods rich in water for fifteen hours; they also had lapses in memory and found it difficult to concentrate.

The National Academy of Sciences suggests that women consume eleven cups of fluid every day (men need about sixteen cups). About eight cups can come from drinks, and the rest from what you eat. Fruits and vegetables are obvious sources (and yummy—

a cup of watermelon contains almost a full cup of water), but many foods, like beans and oatmeal, have at least half a cup.

Don't like plain water? Try iced green tea or sparkling water. One more thing: Avoid using too many caffeinated beverages like coffee or diet soda as part of your water count. Caffeine itself isn't as dehydrating as you may have thought—it only has a diuretic effect if you consume large amounts (more than five hundred milligrams, which equals four or more cups of coffee a day). Even so, it's not good to drink too many caffeinated drinks, as they can make you jittery or interfere with your sleep. Stick with water—it's calorie-free, caffeine-free, and good for you!

REVIVE IN 5!

Sip DIY Designer Water

Don't care for the taste of water? Give it a makeover by adding a splash of fruit juice (I like orange or grapefruit); a tablespoon of chopped crushed berries; or a slice of lemon, lime, or cucumber. For spicier water, stir in a quarter teaspoon of chopped ginger.

Rev Up with a Smart Snack

I need to eat a little something every three to four hours. Typically, I eat breakfast at seven, and by ten I'm ready for a slice of fresh pineapple and a small handful of almonds. For lunch, I'll eat a tuna or turkey sandwich, or grilled-chicken salad, and by three or so a dollop of hummus and some baby carrots, or some fruit and yogurt, hit the spot. Presto—energy up, hunger pangs gone!

Snacking keeps your metabolism revved and is a great way to boost your energy. But not just any snack will do. You need one that's full of nutrients to power you through to your next meal.

As you might have guessed, I recommend whole foods and complex carbs.

Those of you who know me know I'm not much of a calorie counter. But I'll take a guess and say that my snacks fall into the 100- to 200-calorie range. That amount of calories—especially if they come from the right amounts of complex carbs, lean protein, and healthy fats—keeps your metabolism revved, with no tummy growls or energy "blackouts."

10 Favorite Smart Snacks

The most energizing snacks combine healthy carbs and protein (good choices: lean cuts of meat, poultry, fish, eggs, beans, nuts, and low-fat dairy products). Try out the following winning teams for a between-meal pick-me-up. You can even carry most of these healthful snacks with you so you can fuel up on the run.

1. Your favorite fruit with an ounce of cheese or nuts.
2. Half a turkey sandwich on a slice of whole-grain bread, spread with mustard and topped with lettuce and tomato.
3. High-fiber, low-sugar cereal mixed with half a cup of low-fat cottage cheese or yogurt. (Try it—it's good!)
4. Dried fruit and nuts.
5. Air-popped popcorn and a piece of string cheese.
6. Cut-up veggies and two tablespoons of hummus.
7. A baked potato—bake it at home or microwave it at work.
8. Half a cup of cottage cheese mixed with a little chopped-up tomato, carrot, and onion, and sprinkled with cracked black pepper. Spoon it on five or six rye crackers—yum!
9. Natural peanut butter and banana on a rice cake.
10. A small whole-grain pita pocket with hummus and raw veggies.

REVIVE IN 5!

Go Nuts

A small palmful of almonds or walnuts makes the perfect quick pick-me-up, and nuts are much yummier, and more energizing, than an energy drink or candy bar. Nuts' blend of protein, fat, and fiber takes longer to absorb and digest than the simple, fast-burning sugars in sweets or calorie-heavy coffee-shop lattes.

GET A GOOD NIGHT'S SLEEP

I'm an early-to-bed, early-to-rise type—my days are so packed, I am usually fast asleep before the 11 PM news! Most experts agree that we need eight hours of sleep per night—one of its primary functions is to help the brain recover and repair itself. But you may not know that *when* you turn in, and get up, matters too.

It's better for your body to sleep and wake early (from, say, 10 PM to 6 AM) than late (say, 1 AM to 9 AM). The reason: Your body's functions—things like temperature, secretion of hormones, digestion, and other restorative processes—follow a twenty-four-hour cycle linked to its exposure to natural light. When you go to sleep late, and rise late, your body clock gets out of sync. Think of the times you've gone to bed at 3 AM and gotten up at 11 AM the next day. Don't you tend to feel worn down, groggy, and out of sorts? Research suggests that getting just ninety minutes' less sleep—for just one night—can reduce your alertness the next day by more than 30 percent. What's more, a British sleep researcher, Jim Horne, director of the Sleep Research Centre at I
University, says that women need a bit more sleep
about twenty minutes per night. We women tend
more things at once, which means we use more

brains than men tend to do. Because our brains work a bit harder, they need more sleep time to recover.

Try to hit the sack by 10 PM. I know how impossible this may seem—many women use the night hour to do housework or bills, or snatch some time for themselves after an exhausting day of work, social commitments, and family. But think of it this way: Get to bed early, and you're likely to sail through your days—with enough energy for your hectic schedule and yourself!

Can't Sleep? Smart Solutions

Normally, when my head hits the pillow, I'm out like a light, but even I have trouble dropping off sometimes. And when you have trouble getting to sleep, you're draining one of your prime energy sources! Here are some simple solutions to some common sleep problems. If you don't find solutions here, log on to the National Sleep Foundation's website: www.sleepfoundation.org.

- **You worry instead of sleep.** Don't just lie there—get up and go to another part of the house, but leave the lights low or off. Within minutes, your worries should ease, so you can return to bed and fall asleep. Or make a "worry list" in the early evening. Take a few minutes to write down your worries—and possible solutions. That way, come bedtime, you can drift off instead of fret.
- **You watch TV in bed.** Stop! Make your bedroom off limits to any activity except sleep and lovemaking. Don't do paperwork or pay bills in bed, either. You might even consider moving your TV and/or your computer out of your bedroom, to remove temptation.
- **Your partner snores.** This is a tough one, but the solution starts with talking to your partner about the problem. He may have a sleep disorder, such as sleep apnea; gently encourage

him to see a doctor about it. In the meantime, ask your partner to sleep on his side, or invest in a pair of earplugs.

- **There's too much noise (or not enough).** Try to block out unwanted sounds with earplugs, or use "white noise" such as a ceiling fan or an air conditioner or filter. You can also invest in a white-noise machine. If you can't take noise, this will block out disruptive sounds. These methods also provide just enough noise if you can't sleep in total silence.

REVIVE IN 5!

Break Through That Morning Fog

You slept eight hours, but your brain is still fried. The culprit: a phenomenon called sleep inertia. When you first wake up, the parts of your brain that deal with consciousness, called the thalamus and brain stem, start working right away. But the part that handles problem solving and complex thought, called the prefrontal cortex, needs time to get online.

In fact, a University of Colorado–Boulder study found that people who wake up after eight hours of *sound* sleep have more impaired thinking and memory skills than they would after going without sleep for more than twenty-four hours. The topper: For a short period, the effects of sleep inertia may be as bad as or worse than being legally drunk! Further, your supply of fuel (glucose) is nearly empty, and your brain needs a continuous supply of it to function at its best.

The remedy? A bowl of cereal and one cup of coffee. Researchers at Tufts University found that people who ate a serving of oatmeal with half a cup of skim milk received a continuous infusion of glucose, which kept them alert throughout the morning and improved their ability to think. The cuppa? One mug can fight sleep inertia, a University of Pennsylvania study found.

- **You sleep with your pet.** You may love your pet, but animal snuffles and movements can really disrupt your sleep. Could you provide your dog or cat with a bed in your bedroom, instead of sharing your bed? Think about it—you'll have more energy and love to give him or her the next day!
- **You have allergies.** Whatever you're allergic to, keep it clean. Your house and bedroom, that is. Vacuum and dust once a week, and wash sheets and blankets (and even your pillow) once a week in hot water. Use a dehumidifier to help prevent the accumulation of mold spores. Encase your pillow in a plastic cover under your pillowcase to keep dust mites from interfering with your sleep and allergy or asthma symptoms. Crack the windows and doors, too—increasing a room's airflow is one of the best ways to reduce dust mites according to a study in the *Journal of Allergy and Clinical Immunology.*

Power Up with a Power Nap

I've never been a napper. But now that I've hit fifty, I find that when I wake up at 2 AM to pee, it can take me an hour to get back to sleep, which can sap my energy the next day. On those days, a catnap really hits the spot, helping me feel more rested, positive, and alert. My experience is backed by many studies that show that naps, like nighttime sleep, enhance the ability to process information and learn. A twenty-minute nap can clear your head and boost your energy when you're running a sleep deficit. But don't make it a habit to nap during the day to make up for lack of nighttime sleep. The body uses those eight hours to repair itself, and if you nap too long and too often, you'll mess up your ability to sleep at night.

RECHARGE WITH EXERCISE

Scout's honor: I exercise just thirty minutes a day. But that half hour does so much good for my body, mind, and spirit—and those benefits translate into my sky-high energy levels! The "bounce" that exercise gives me will work for you, too.

Regular exercise has long been known to increase vitality. In one study published in 2008, researchers at the University of Georgia found that inactive folks who normally complained of fatigue increased their energy by 20 percent—and reduced their fatigue by as much as 65 percent—when they participated in regular, low-intensity exercise.

Why does exercise energize? Well, regular workouts train your body to use oxygen and glucose—its main sources of fuel—more efficiently. They also condition your heart and lungs, which energizes you further—your cells are getting more oxygen, remember?

I know how tough it can be to get to the gym, or to take your daily stroll, when all you want to do is curl up on the couch. But remember this mantra: To get energy, you need to expend it—and sooner than you think, you'll be living proof of that!

REBOOT WITH ENERGY BREAKS

We all know what coffee breaks and cigarette breaks are (unfortunately!). But how many of us take an energy break? I don't mean taking an hour for yourself, as wonderful as this is. I'm talking sixty to ninety *seconds*.

Just for today, try this: Every hour, on the hour, whether you're at home or at work, get up off that rear. Stand up, swing your arms, stretch your arms over your head, bound up or down a flight of stairs, take a deep breath. (Go on—do it right now!) Bathe those cells in the oxygen they crave. Get that blood pumping!

You'll be amazed at how dramatically that tiny sliver of time can refresh and renew your body and mind.

The science behind the energy break is pretty simple: Moving around stimulates your circulation. Good circulation is essential for energy because blood transports oxygen and nutrients—fuel for your cells—to your muscles and your brain.

Think of an hourly energy break as a little oasis for your body and mind. When you stand up, stretch, and take a few deep breaths, you take a mini vacation from the things that keep your body and mind in park, like your computer, e-mail and voice mail, or those less-than-positive clients or co-workers. And lest you forget, set your watch every hour to remind you, or jot it on your scheduling software. Or simply stick a Post-it note on your computer screen.

REVIVE IN 5!

A Stretch to Open Your Heart

A great yoga teacher, B. K. S. Iyengar, always says: "If you keep your armpits open, you won't get depressed." While it sounds wacky, he's really talking about opening the chest and shoulders and keeping your head in midline, which allows your breath to flow freely.

Think about it: When you feel blue, your posture shows it. Your head hangs down, your chest sinks in, and your shoulders round forward. To get your oxygen flowing, open yourself up—to oxygen and positivity—with this simple exercise: Sit tall in a chair with your knees together and your feet flat on the floor. Clasp your hands behind your neck, with your elbows up and back. Lean back so that your back is slightly arched and your armpits are open. Lift and open your chest as you look at the ceiling. Feel the stretch through your clavicle and your sternum. Hold, breathing normally, for ten seconds, and then repeat. Now you should feel refreshed and revitalized!

Take energy breaks on long car trips, too. Get out of the car and treat yourself to some fresh air and a stretch. Ditto when you watch television or talk on the phone—I actually do stretches and knee bends while I do phone interviews. After a while, these mini breaks will become a habit, burn extra calories, and your energy levels will reflect it.

ZAP STRESS

Yes, I get stressed—I'm human! But because stress is a major energy drain, I'm very careful not to let it get its hooks in me. I'm a look-on-the-bright-side type of person, so when stress tries to poke its nose into my day, I try to remember that while it may be a part of life, I can control how I react to it. Attitude—it makes all the difference.

Science knows the toll that chronic stress (the kind that never ends, like a long commute, money worries, or a toxic relationship) takes on mind and body. Low but chronic levels of stress wear away your energy, so if you don't bring it under control, all you'll want to do is stay in bed, with the covers over your head.

Chronic stress is different from short-term stress—the kind that has a beginning and end (think of a fender-bender in a parking lot). Under short-term stress, your body releases the hormone cortisol. When released, this fight-or-flight hormone increases the fat and sugar in your bloodstream, to get your brain and muscles a quick burst of energy to react. After the stress has passed, your body returns to normal.

Under *chronic* stress, however, your body pumps out cortisol constantly—and such long-term exposure to elevated cortisol wears you down and leaves you vulnerable to colds or chronic conditions from diabetes to cancer.

The first thing I do when I'm stressed is focus on my breathing.

Deep breaths—in through the nose, out through my lips, like I'm whistling. Now try breathing in through your nose and exhaling through your nose. This really does focus and calm me. Deep breathing increases the oxygen in your bloodstream, which slows your heart rate, lowers your blood pressure, and relaxes your muscles, counteracting the fight-or-flight response.

Chronic stress is epidemic in our society, especially for women. While it's important to make time for an hour, or weekend, to blow off its effects, it's equally important to short-circuit stress throughout the day. That's why, throughout this book, I've created almost-instant stress busters (look for the tips titled "Revive in 5"), plus a few "Peace Pockets" to tuck into your day. And if one doesn't suit you, try another—we're all different, and find different ways to find peace and positivity. The important thing is to consciously take a minute or two of peace, several times a day. Such a tiny slice of time, but such huge benefits for your mood and energy level!

PEACE POCKET

Take a Meditation Walk
Head out for a quiet early-morning walk or lace up your sneakers on your lunch break. This is a ramble, not a brisk walk! Walk in a peaceful place if you can, where there is some nature and quiet.

EMBRACE POSITUDE!
Your mood has a direct impact on your energy. When you're in a low mood, your energy is low. When your mood is high, your energy follows. That's why I try, always, to focus on the good in any situation. Staying positive allows you to take action, and I'm all about taking action to either enjoy life or improve it!

At the end of the day, *positive thinking* is thinking in ways that reduce stress, boost your mood, and take away worry and fear. (In fact, that's a lot of what cognitive behavioral therapy is based on—you learn to change the way you think to deal with life on life's terms.)

Yesterday is gone; tomorrow isn't here yet. All we have is today. When you embrace positude, you know, really *know*, what a gift *today* is. Sixteen waking hours to do the things that give us joy, and to try things that might; to explore who we are and what we want; to offer our help to others; to experience and learn from the gamut of human emotions—joy and loss, happiness and anger—and to accept people, and situations, the way they are, not as we wish them to be. And if today is less than perfect, well, so be it; there's always tomorrow, that fresh start, that clean slate.

Positude is like a plant, and our choices are the ways to care for it. Do we appreciate and celebrate the good in our lives—our families, friends, health, talents? That's the sunlight that encourages the seed to reach up and out of the darkness. Do we connect with others with kindness, and care as much for their welfare as for our own? There's the water it needs to flourish. Meet adversity with courage, clarity, and calm? We've pulled the weeds to encourage vitality and growth. And in life, as in rosebushes or tomato plants, growth is the name of the game!

The power of positive thinking isn't new—but research into its power continues. Some of the newest research is from Barbara Fredrickson, PhD, author of *Positivity* and a professor at the Positive Emotions and Psychophysiology Lab (the PEPLab!) at the University of North Carolina–Chapel Hill. Dr. Fredrickson's "Broaden-and-Build" theory explains how increasing positive emotions creates an upward spiral that leads to more positive emotions as well as more creative and flexible thinking, resilience, and a sense of purpose. Her research further suggests that we need to experience three positive emotions to every negative emotion. The point isn't to banish negative emotions completely, nor to strive for a constant state of euphoria. The goal—always a worthy one—is balance.

TAP INTO NATURE'S ENERGY

Although I've lived just outside Washington, DC, for twenty-five years now, I'm a California girl at heart—I love the sun and natural beauty. So I've always felt what scientists continue to prove: When you commune with nature, your mental and emotional energy skyrocket.

Several recent studies, all published in the *Journal of Environmental Psychology*, concluded that exposure to nature is linked to greater vitality, which the researchers described as feeling alive—enthusiastic, happy, alert, and full of energy.

In one of these studies, people who strolled outdoors reported increased vitality, while those who walked indoors saw no change. A few of the other studies looked at volunteers' activities during a two-week period and found that being exposed to nature, and even just going outside to experience sunlight and fresh air, boosted vitality. (In a few of the studies, participants didn't even have to go outside—just thinking about being outside pepped them up!)

Here's another benefit nature grants us: Outdoor air contains a high balance of negative ions (molecules with a negative electrical charge), which may increase your body's intake of oxygen and levels of a feel-good brain chemical called serotonin, according to Michael Terman, PhD, director of the Center for Light Treatment and Biological Rhythms at New York Presbyterian Hospital. Odorless, tasteless, and invisible, negative ions are plentiful in natural settings such as mountains, waterfalls, and beaches. Once they reach our bloodstream, they're believed to produce biochemical reactions that increase levels of serotonin.

You don't have to live next to breathtaking vistas to experience the energizing power of nature. Spread a blanket on your lawn to watch the sun rise, or set. Walk in a gentle summer shower. Dig in your garden. Stroll in the woods. If you're a city dweller, head to the park and soak up some sun. Nature can be found almost anywhere, so get outside and meet it.

PEACE POCKET

Watch, or Feed, the Birds

Finally—a use for that old set of binoculars! Dust them off, take them to work, and when you're stressed, find a quiet spot to observe the world above your head for a few minutes. Watch the birds sing, scold, feed their young, fight. You don't need a bird-watching guide, just a sense of wonder. At home, step outside, armed with a few pieces of stale bread or birdseed, and let them come to you.

ENERGY MAKEOVER!

MICHELLE RACE, 39
HOMETOWN: TUCSON, ARIZONA
OCCUPATION: 9-1-1 DISPATCHER

I recently received an e-mail from Michelle, whose major energy zapper is her schedule—she works from 2 AM to noon four days a week. "I love my job, but my work schedule is sapping my energy," she wrote. "I go to bed at 4 PM, *try* to sleep eight hours (although it's usually more like six), and set my alarm for midnight. I can get very groggy at work!"

Near the end of the week, when Michelle is really exhausted, she'll "sleep in," which for her means she gets up at 6 or 7 AM instead of midnight.

Michelle also deals with tremendous stress. "As gratifying as my job is, it is also stressful," she explains. "Every day, I deal with callers in some of the most desperate moments of their lives. Although dispatchers are taught basic ways to cope with the stress we face, it does occasionally follow me home."

Michelle's overall work environment isn't the most energizing, either. "Basically, all we can do is sit!" she writes. "We're plugged into a console via a headset and must remain at our desks for our ten- to twelve-hour workdays. We get ten-minute breaks every two to three hours, and I try to use mine to take a lap or two around our parking lot, just to get my blood circulating and fresh oxygen into my lungs. It definitely helps—the dispatching room is dark, so that shot of sun helps revive me. But I can't get out there all the time, and when I don't do a lap I definitely feel it."

Michelle and her fellow dispatchers must sit at their desks to eat, too. "And eat we do!" says Michelle. "Food runs for burritos, burgers, and pizza occur just about every shift." Michelle admits that her weakness is those sugary, chocolatey coffee drinks—"I think I get more of a jolt from the sugar in them than the caffeine!" Unfortunately, after she drinks it, she'll "crash" and get tired again—which leaves her little energy for exercise. "I've probably put on twenty pounds since I started this job—and the extra weight makes me feel tired and sluggish. If I lost some, I would feel much more energetic, I think."

Michelle tries not to let the stress and sedentary nature of her job get to her, "but I am *tired*. I feel completely drained on my workdays and have lost my motivation to do much on my days off."

But Michelle has begun to fight that negativity. She's tried to lay off the food, and just signed up for a boot camp class with some girlfriends from work. When that's over, her next ambition is to begin tennis lessons. "I'm a pretty upbeat person overall and, luckily, have lots of emotional support—my family in New York State and great friends in my area—but I definitely need to take control and get my energy back. SOS!"

Well, hats off to you, Michelle—you're one of the heroes! Let's pump up your energy so you can enjoy life outside of work.

As a shift worker, I'm sure you know that odd work hours disrupt your body's natural rhythms. It sounds like you've established a routine, which "trains" your body to know when to be alert and when to sleep, but what keeps you from sleeping eight solid hours?

When you're a shift worker, it's important to keep to the same bedtime and wake-time schedule. If light and noise disturb your sleep, wear an eye mask to block sunlight or splurge on a white-noise machine to eliminate outside sounds. And while it's not a good idea to sleep in on weekends (you want to train your body, remember?), there's nothing wrong with taking a fifteen-minute catnap to rejuvenate. Finally, when it's time to change your shift, ask if you can "schedule your shift clockwise"—that is, so that your new shift would start later than your current one.

About that coffee drink: It's fine to drink coffee at the start of your shift, but why not switch to iced herbal green tea a few times a week? It's so good for you and it won't give you the jitters. When you do drink coffee, stop four hours before your shift ends—and definitely swap that calorie-laden coffee drink for a decaffeinated "skinny" latte or other low-calorie, low-sugar beverage. In your line of work, you just don't need the crash—from either caffeine or sugar!

Those "food runs" must be tough to resist—I love the burritos in Tucson! (I went to the University of Arizona.) But if you want to lose weight and regain your energy, you have to stand firm. It's time to scour cookbooks and the Internet for recipes for familiar favorites that contain good amounts of healthy carbs and proteins. Why not cook up a batch of low-fat chicken burritos or rice and beans on the weekends, so you can take them to work? Add a piece of fruit, and if you need a snack, opt for sliced veggies and a low-calorie dip. Or snack on a couple of hard-boiled eggs—the whites provide plenty of protein. Portion control is important, too. When you sit for ten to twelve hours, your body doesn't need large amounts of calories. Maybe you can even inspire some of your co-workers to do the same, and you can motivate one another.

It's great that you take those laps around the parking lot— nothing can refresh, recharge, and de-stress like a brisk, ten-minute walk, and the sunshine will boost your mood and help fight that on-the-job grogginess. I'd encourage you to get in at least two of them per shift—you can eat anytime, so get your meal in before or after your laps. If you simply can't, do my afternoon stretching routine on your breaks.

Your biggest ally in your battle to regain your energy is your positive attitude. You know you have the power to change what holds you back—so many people don't, and the fact that you do makes all the difference!

That boot camp, and those tennis lessons, will do more than boost your energy. They'll also help you blow off the stress of your work and remind you that there's life outside the dispatch room. What's more, you'll learn new skills and set yourself challenges that engage both your body and your mind. You've even got a built-in cheering section—support is so important! Keep that can-do frame of mind, but don't think you have to do it all. Move, breathe, eat, and sleep well, and call on others when you need them. You'll find that those extra pounds—and that stress—will melt away!

CHAPTER 5

Change Your Outlook, Recharge Your Life

People have called me the Energizer Bunny 'cause I just keep going and going. But they don't just notice my energy...they tell me they feel my *positive* energy!

While physical stamina is an important part of energy, it's equally important that this energy come from a happy, positive outlook. Why clutter your mind with negative thoughts when you can choose to fill it with good ones? That's right, you can *choose* to be happy, *choose* to put a bounce in your step, *choose* to focus on what's good in life. As I always say, attitude is everything!

Your attitude is shaped by your thoughts. Positive thoughts—*most people mean well, most situations turn out for the best*—lead to a positive attitude. A positive attitude leads to positive action. Note that word: *action*. If, on the other hand, your mind whispers a constant refrain of *What's the use?*—your behavior will reflect it. You may skip the gym, binge on junk, start smoking again, stew instead of sleep, or zone out in front of the TV or computer. The resulting stress, self-pity, emptiness, or fatigue will suck the juice right out of you. Negativity is like quicksand—the deeper you sink, the harder it is to move.

Maybe you've bought into the idea that positive thinking is silly and delusional. Being the optimist that I am, I prefer to see it as practical. People who search for the positive in a negative event aren't delusional. They're *resilient*. Rather than shake their fist at the sky, they pick themselves up and go on. Seems pretty practical to me!

I can't promise that if you think positive, your life will magically become perfect. What I can promise is that you'll feel less stressed and more energetic.

The suggestions that follow can help you begin to see the glass as half full. Start with the ones that seem easiest to you; as one becomes a habit, try another. Also, expect some setbacks. Old habits die hard, so if you slip into negative thinking now and

---

REVIVE IN 5!

The Positive-Thinking Nightcap

Each night before bed, review your day and ask yourself these three questions.

1. **At any point today, did I choose to take the positive view?** Congratulate yourself—well done!

2. **At any point today, did I slip into negative thinking?** Play a game with yourself: How would an optimist see this situation? Then try to flip those negative thoughts into a more positive view.

3. **What shall I look forward to tomorrow?** Pick something, no matter how small—your morning cup of coffee, a hug from your honey, or wearing the new lipstick you picked up today. Practice makes perfect—the more you look for something to look forward to, the more you'll find!

then, let it go and start anew. With practice, patience, and commitment, you *can* train yourself to accentuate the positive. Before long, your self-talk will change. Your attitude will brighten. And your get-up-and-go, which got up and went a long time ago, will come back.

LOOK FOR THE LAUGHS

Think back to your last genuine belly laugh—an outburst that had you doubled over, shaking helplessly, tears streaming, ab muscles begging for mercy. Well, that laugh didn't just change your outlook—it changed your body, too. You tensed, then released, the muscles in your face and throughout your body. Your circulation sped up, and you breathed faster, which sent more oxygen to your tissues. Sounds a lot like a good stretch, doesn't it?

Researchers have studied the possible benefits of laughter on our health for decades now, and the findings are intriguing, if yet to be proven beyond a doubt. To give just one example, laughter may reduce the damaging effects of inflammation, a process linked to heart disease, diabetes, and other chronic conditions.

Four Fascinating Facts About Laughter

1. Studies have pinpointed eighteen different kinds of smiles. The most common is the smile of enjoyment.
2. We use thirteen muscles to smile, but forty-seven to frown.
3. To make one wrinkle, you have to smile nearly 250,000 times.
4. According to a study by German psychologist Michael Titze, in the 1950s people laughed an average of eighteen minutes a day. Today that's down to four to six minutes a day.

What is known is that laughter produces a chemical reaction that instantly boosts mood, reduces pain, and eases stress. A study by researchers at Stanford University traced this reaction to a region called the nucleus accumbens, which rewards behaviors such as eating, sex, and laughter with the release of the brain chemical dopamine, a natural opiate. Belly laughter also empties your lungs of more air than they take in—an effect similar to deep breathing, which sends more oxygen-enriched blood and nutrients throughout the body.

But you don't need studies to convince you that a burst of genuine laughter feels good—that when you feel blue or stressed, it refreshes and re-energizes. My personal view is that laughter that stems from goodhearted humor is the best laughter "medicine."

That said, everyone's sense of humor is different, and what makes me laugh may not work for you. So seek out the comedians, movies, jokes, and books that you *know* make you laugh. When I need a laugh, I'll flip on the tube and look for reruns of *I Love Lucy* or *Seinfeld*. And I love when my daughters find a funny clip on YouTube—that way, we all get to laugh together!

Whatever flips your laughter switch, involve other people—studies show that we laugh more when we're with others. Hang around funny people. Soak up their natural energy. Trade some jokes. Before long, you'll laugh more, and drag less!

LEND A HAND

As a member of the President's Council on Physical Fitness and Sports, I've traveled to schools all across America. I'll arrive at a school with a boom box, blast the music, and lead one big exercise jam session! We have push-up and sit-up contests, do jumping jacks, and generally have a great time. I love to see the smiles on these kids' faces! That feeling of connection, the sense that I've made a difference in someone's life—those positive feelings stay with me a long time.

In other words, I'm feeling that so-called helper's high. People who volunteer regularly—an hour or two a week—tend to live longer, have lower rates of depression, and recover more quickly from illness. In fact, states with high volunteerism have lower rates of mortality and incidence of heart disease.

But why do we feel so good when we help others? Whether you volunteer at your child's school, your community food bank, an animal shelter, or a hospice, you put the welfare of others before your own, however briefly. Further, when you make a positive difference in the world—teach a troubled teen to read, pack food for distribution at a local food bank, even donate blood—you reap what you have sown: emotional energy and positivity.

Researchers theorize that when you volunteer, you have the opportunity to walk in other people's shoes, which makes you

REVIVE IN 5!

Volunteer a Kind Word

Sometimes I call one of my fans out of the blue just to say hello and cheer them on (or sometimes cheer them up!). They can't believe it's me, but my voice gives me away. That fifteen-minute phone call leaves me feeling charged all day!

You can make the same kind of impact in someone's day, just by being you. Giving someone even a minute or two of your time or attention can make a big impact in the life of someone in need. If you can't volunteer in the traditional sense, "volunteer" a word of comfort or encouragement to someone who needs it every day. You might also send a card to someone who is struggling with personal or health troubles.

appreciate the gifts in your own life. A 1988 article in *Psychology Today,* which called this phenomenon the helper's high, analyzed two surveys of thirty-two hundred women who volunteered on a regular basis. The article described a physical response from volunteer work similar to the results of vigorous exercise or meditation.

If you're not sure how to get involved, here are a few ideas to get you started:

- Donate blood.
- Do yard work for an elderly or disabled neighbor.
- Join the local literacy association and teach people to read.
- Join the PTA at your child's school.
- Coach a kids' soccer or softball team.
- Volunteer at a local animal shelter.
- Cook or serve meals for your community homeless shelter.

Positive energy comes from the knowledge that you've made a difference in your tiny part of the planet.

STOP NEGATIVE THOUGHTS NOW

I try not to have negative thoughts—they use up valuable mental and emotional energy. Plus, I've seen the way negative thoughts diminish and deflate those who indulge in them. I've known many smart, gorgeous women who had everything going for them— looks, brains, talent. But they just couldn't stop with the "what-ifs" and the "I should haves" or the "I'll nevers." They thought themselves out of happiness and success.

Worry is like a hole in your gas tank—unfixed, it will drain your precious energy and you'll sputter to a stop. But you can plug that leak in a second. Simply accept life as it is, in this moment.

Here's an easy way to banish those negative thoughts for good.

It's called thought-stopping, and it's used by therapists to help clients who think themselves into self-defeating behaviors. With this technique, you focus on a negative thought, and then interrupt it with the word "*Stop.*" (You'll need to raise your voice a bit, so make sure you pick a private place.) The more you practice, the better it will work, and once you master it you can use it anytime a negative thought tries to take up space in your head. Here's how to proceed.

1. List your most stressful thoughts, from most stressful to least stressful. Then, armed with a timer (your watch will do, too), settle into a comfy chair in a quiet, *private* place.
2. Start with your least stressful thought. Close your eyes and think about the stressful or negative thought. Imagine yourself in the situation that typically triggers the thought. Really get into it. If you feel yourself begin to get angry or anxious, let it happen.
3. Now you're ready to stop the thought: Set the timer for three minutes and again focus on your negative thought. When the timer sounds, shout "Stop!" If you want, stand up, snap your fingers, or clap your hands to "punctuate" the word.
4. Close your eyes again and take several slow, deep breaths through your nose. If the negative thought returns, shout "Stop!" again.

PEACE POCKET

Look at Photos from a Happy Time

Pull out snapshots from your photo album of good times with family or friends—your youngest child's first day of kindergarten, a family vacation, a friend's wedding. Lose yourself in the happy memory of that occasion.

5. Repeat these steps until the thought stops when you shout. Then repeat them using a normal tone of voice. When a normal tone stops the thought, whisper. Over time, you can just say "Stop" in your head. Repeat the technique with any other negative thoughts, working your way up your list to the most stressful.

THE ATTITUDE MAKEOVER

There are beauty makeovers. Fashion makeovers. House makeovers. Why not give your attitude a makeover, too? A positive outlook begins with a positive thought. The "before" list shows common examples of negative thoughts. The "after" list shows the positive, yet realistic alternatives.

BEFORE	AFTER
I'm a total failure.	I didn't meet my goal this time. I'll figure out why and try again.
My entire life is a mess.	Things are tough right now, but I've been through rough times before. I'll make it through.
If I can't do it perfectly, there's no point in doing it.	I can strive for perfection, but under these circumstances a good job is good enough.
She walked right by and didn't say hello. She must not like me.	She's been friendly before. Perhaps she has a lot on her mind.

I'll never lose this weight.	I've lost weight before, when I worked out and ate right. If I do those things, I will lose weight again.
I'm a bad daughter—I should call my mother more.	Mom pushes my buttons, so it's okay to take care of myself and call her once a week.
Why even try? I'll just fail anyway.	Why not try? If I fail, who cares? At least I tried my best.

GET GRATEFUL

I have a happy, healthy family, a group of girlfriends that I love, and a large extended family to whom I'm very connected. I have the career I always dreamed of (and worked for!), my health, and my faith, thanks to my grandma. I know how fortunate I am, and I give thanks every day. When I stop to appreciate the good in my life, gratitude sprouts in my heart like a seed—any stress or negativity is washed clean away.

People who feel gratitude have more vitality and optimism and suffer less stress than the population as a whole, studies show.

REVIVE IN 5!

There's Energy in Numbers!

Every time I'm around my daughters' lacrosse team and their parents, my energy rises to a new level. Stay close to people who love and support one another 100 percent—they'll rev up your energy in no time!

These results hold even when researchers factor out age, health, and income.

What that means is that feelings of gratitude don't come more easily to the young, rich, or healthy. There are countless folks who don't seem to have much to be thankful for—people with a serious illness, or who lose their home in a fire or natural disaster— who overflow with gratitude. *It all depends on your perspective—how you look at human nature and the world.* And if that perspective is less than positive, it's within your power to change it.

So if it's been a while since you counted your blessings, here are two ways to start.

1. **Jot down the gifts in your life.** In a notebook, on your computer, on a board with erasable markers—keep a running log of the gifts in your life. (Get your family to join in!) When you actually write down your blessings, you have black-and-white "evidence" of your gratitude. Plus, it works. In a study of college students, those who kept weekly gratitude journals exercised more regularly, felt better about their lives as a whole, and maintained greater optimism about the future.

2. **Thank your challenges and obstacles.** Start to say "thank you," either silently or aloud, each time you're presented with a difficult person or situation. Then find the ways in which this person or situation can ultimately benefit you. For instance, your mother-in-law can help you develop patience and compassion. Even a situation as scary as a layoff can be a gift in disguise: a fresh start.

EXPLORE THE WORLD AROUND YOU

In an uncertain and chaotic world, routines make life predictable and more productive. Routines also make life safe, which is a double-edged sword. When we feel too safe, our routine can feel more like a rut, one of the biggest energy drainers there is.

When you're stuck in a rut, you have to break out—and recent research confirms that new experiences infuse you with energy. Novelty and challenge are key components of satisfaction, which generates vitality, according to Gregory Berns, MD, a neuroscientist at Emory University in Atlanta and the author of *Satisfaction: The Science of Finding True Fulfillment.* Says Dr. Berns, "We've known that when people try something new, the brain's reward chemical, dopamine, is released. But there's an added benefit: dopamine is also a motivating chemical that gears us up to do more."

In other words, if you take an art class at the local community college, you may get fired up to take on a new project at home or at work, which creates an upward positive spiral of energy.

Look for small ways to introduce more novelty into your life, today. Maybe one day you'll run a marathon, or open that business you've always dreamed about, or take a trip around the world. But the first step to turning those new, brain- and soul-energizing dreams into reality is to start small, and start *now*. For example, you might brush your teeth with or hold your fork in your opposite hand, or rearrange your bedroom furniture. If you take your walk along a path that splits, you can take the fork you've never tried. Learn to play a new game—bridge, poker, chess—or play a video game with your kids and accept that they will beat the pants off you. You could also thrill your taste buds with a cuisine you've never tried—Indian, Middle Eastern, Ethiopian—or enroll in an adult-education class at the local community college. Choose a course that truly excites you—learn the history of music or art, a new language, photography, writing.

I've often said that there are two types of people—those with backbones, and those with wishbones. People with backbones dream, and then turn their dreams into action. People with wishbones dream, too...but their dreams stay trapped in their heads. To let those dreams take flight, shake things up! Once you do that, you're on the road to becoming the more positive and energetic person you were born to be.

DO A DRESS REHEARSAL FOR FAILURE

Failure gets a bad rap. You know that line in *The Empire Strikes Back*, when Yoda says, "Do, or do not—there is no try"? I have to disagree with this wise old Jedi Master. There *is* such a thing as "try," and it balances precariously between "success" and "failure."

To expend blood, sweat, and tears—*energy*—to achieve your aspirations, you need to believe you can succeed. But you also need to be comfortable with the idea that you might fail. You have to believe that even if you fail, the energy you put into the attempt to succeed is not wasted. To not try unless you know beyond a doubt that you will succeed is to shortchange yourself. To embrace the possibility of failure is to be liberated from expectation. Only then—when you've "baked" the possibility of failure into your pie in the sky—will you have the chance of the pure joy that "try" can bring.

Visualizing yourself succeeding in your mind's eye really can, and does, work. I've spent a lot of time around professional athletes, so I know this from personal experience. To give just one example: My husband's little sister, Tracy Austin, visualized winning the U.S. Open—and she did it in 1979, and again in 1981!

Positive thinking can play a role in helping you land a job, improve your health, or turn a bad relationship around. Still, if you confront the fear, honestly, openly, and head-on—and don't get the results you want—that's okay! No matter how ardently you focus on success, failure is still an option.

Failure terrifies most people. In fact, our culture frowns on it. *We're Americans, darn it, and Americans don't fail!* Baloney. More people should fail more, because failure would be proof that they've actually gotten off their duffs and tried!

If you're terrified by the idea of failure, try this visualization. See yourself try for what you want—to fit in that cute little black dress, write a novel, run a marathon, or start your own business. Whatever it is, visualize yourself taking the steps necessary to achieve that dream. See yourself rising at dawn to train. Designing a website for your business and placing cold calls to potential clients. Sitting at your keyboard and pounding away as your story and characters come alive.

Now see yourself fail. You're dropping out of the marathon after six miles. Those would-be clients are politely declining your product or service.

Then see yourself go on after that failure. What do you do? Visualize it exactly, right down to the expression on your face. Well, maybe first you shed some tears or throw yourself on your bed, kicking and screaming. But after that—see yourself after the marathon on the car ride home, wrapped in friends' and family's love and support, or dialing one more client.

Perform this visualization until you know *exactly* how you'd react in the event of failure. More often than not, you'll come up with ways to try again. And after each run-through, remember this quote, which has variously been attributed to both Albert Einstein and Thomas Edison: "I have not failed. I've just found 10,000 ways that won't work."

When you risk leaving your personal comfort zone and test your boundaries, there is a possibility that you could fail. But you know what? It's okay to fail. What is not okay is not to try. Nothing in my life prepared me more for my successes than my failures—and there have been plenty of them!

In 1984, I tried thirty-five times to get the producer of the *Today* show on the phone. I wanted to pitch him my idea of being the fitness expert on the show, an idea that had never been tried before. Every single time I called, the producer's secretary said, "Sorry, he's not in right now." But I wouldn't give up—and finally, on the thirty-sixth try, he took my call! He loved my enthusiasm and passion for what I did, and agreed to let me do a two-day fitness series. Well, after that series ran, I got ten thousand letters in one week…more than Willard Scott got that week! I'd pictured myself being on that show—and I got there. Pure determination and persistence paid off for me, and they will for you, too. Just keep trying, and eventually, you will succeed!

When you are at peace with the possibility of failure, you'll find a well of untapped energy with which to pursue success.

BE HERE NOW!

Our lives whiz by at ninety miles an hour—and all too often, we're not even at the wheel. There aren't enough hours in the day to accomplish what we must, let alone what we want. We have little time to react to what life pitches, and even less to reflect on it. We're moving so fast, it's hard to know who we are and what we want. This frantic pace leads to stress and a vicious circle. Stress drains our energy. Low in physical, mental, or emotional energy, we become less effective, which means we're less able to use our time efficiently, which leads to more stress. The more stress we experience, the less energy we generate; the less energy we generate, the harder it is to manage stress.

As strange as it sounds, the solution to this high-speed, low-energy lifestyle is to *slow down* and learn to live in the moment. One technique we can use is called *mindfulness*. Mindfulness goes back to the time of the spiritual teacher Buddha, who believed that we should neither look back at the past nor anticipate the future. When we stay in the present, in the here and now, we're on the path to inner peace.

While mindfulness is often a part of formal meditation, you can use mindfulness anytime, anyplace—as you sweep the kitchen floor, stand in line at the supermarket deli, or take a shower. All that is required is that you focus on what you're doing, moment by moment. You don't pass judgment; you simply observe.

While mindfulness is a simple technique, it isn't always easy. Often, we're so frantically busy that our bodies and minds run on autopilot. Mindfulness keeps us firmly in the here and now.

You can try mindfulness right now, as you read this book. Mindfulness in this situation might sound like this: *I'm sitting in the family room reading a book while my husband and children watch TV. I feel the weight of the book in my hands, and the smoothness of the cover on my fingers. I am on page 87 right now. I am reading about mindfulness. I hear my family laugh at a funny line. There's still enough light coming through the window that I only have the one lamp beside me turned on. I can smell the vanilla-scented candle I lit this afternoon. I feel very comfortable and content in this chair.*

Continue to observe and report on your thoughts, feelings, sensory impressions, and the world around you until your mind slows down and your stress drains away.

The tiny bit of energy you expend to cultivate mindfulness is far less than all the energy you waste on life's stresses and distractions. Once you begin to cultivate mindfulness, you can renew your vitality and reclaim your life. As mindfulness expert Jon Kabat-Zinn says, "The real meditation is your life, and how you inhabit it moment by moment."

UNPLUG FROM YOUR TV

I love TV. How could I not? I'm usually *on* TV! In fact, my family and I love to watch certain shows together, like *American Idol*. But can you believe the average American watches TV for about five hours a day? Wow! That's pretty sobering, because research suggests that being glued to the tube is linked to weight gain and unhappiness, which are both serious energy drainers. However, a recent study proves that when people do peel themselves away from the tube, they move more, do more, and feel better.

In this study, researchers at the University of Vermont had twenty people cut their daily TV viewing in half, which gave them an extra two hours a day. With that extra free time, they did things like play board games with their kids, housework, and walk the dog. Some even signed up for yoga classes. Regardless of how they used this extra, non-TV time, they burned an average of 120 more calories a day than a control group that watched the tube for five hours a day. That's good for weight loss, of course, but clearly they found a reserve of newfound energy that they used to connect with the world around them and experience pleasure. Remember—positivity breeds energy.

REVIVE IN 5!

When All Seems Lost, Make Your Bed

Many women have told me that they dislike coming home to an unmade bed—those wrinkled sheets are like the last thumbs-down on a bad day. If you can relate, smooth those sheets, pat that comforter, and plump those pillows, even if you plan to mess them up again in an hour. You'll create order out of chaos, and do one small thing to make your world a little brighter. Already made your bed? Clean out the kitchen junk drawer.

I don't mean to suggest that you cut out TV completely—just cut back, the way you might on chocolate chip cookies. There are a few simple ways to do that.

For example, don't reach for the remote unless you're tuning in for a specific show, or use your TiVo or DVR to record so you can watch it later. Some people turn on the TV in the morning, or the second they get home from work, and turn it off only when it's time for bed. It becomes "background music" for their lives! So keep it off unless you plan to actually sit down and watch. If you don't turn it on, you can't get sucked in.

If there's a show you just can't miss, use your two hours to watch that. If you don't use your two-hour limit, "bank" the other hour for an extra-long movie or the big football game.

Even though you'll be watching TV less, get active during commercial breaks—it's an easy way to slip some extra, energy-generating movement into your day. Most hour-long TV shows pack in twenty minutes of commercials. Use those minutes to stretch, or hop on your cardio machine. (I do this when I watch a college basketball game with my husband—he jumps on the bike, I jump on the treadmill!) Do triceps dips off the couch, or do tummy tighteners—pull your knees to your chest ten times as you sit on the edge of the couch. You can even throw your yoga mat on the floor in front of the TV and do a few sets of crunches.

I'm not saying that you should never watch TV or keep up with the news of the day—just be mindful of how much the tube is on. In a way, you might think of TV the way you think of junk food: fine in moderation, but not as a steady diet.

TRY ONE (OR MORE!) OF THESE EASY, RESEARCH-TESTED HAPPINESS BOOSTS

Recently, a group of positive psychology researchers led by the pioneer of happiness psychology, Dr. Martin E. P. Seligman of the University of Pennsylvania, recruited men and women to help test new exercises designed to increase happiness. Almost six hundred men and women volunteered.

The researchers randomly assigned the volunteers one of six exercises, periodically assessing their symptoms of both happiness and depression. Regardless of their assigned exercise, volunteers were asked to do it for just one week. However, they had to complete follow-up tests after completing the exercise.

The exercises were:

- **Three good things in life.** Each night of the week, write down three things that went well that day and why.
- **Using signature strengths in new ways.** Identify your personal strengths, and use at least one in a new way every day for the week.
- **Gratitude visit.** Over the next week, write and deliver a letter of gratitude to someone you have not properly thanked.
- **You at your best.** Write about a time you were at your best, and reflect each night for the next week on your personal strengths that made that time your best.
- **Identify signature strengths.** Identify your personal signature strengths.
- **Early memories.** Write about your earliest memories every night for a week. This exercise was a "placebo," included to compare the results in this group with those of the groups who completed the "real" exercises.

These researchers checked in with these folks by e-mail after a week, a month, three months, and six months. At the end of six months, the researchers found:

- The "Three Good Things" and "Using Signature Strengths" exercises boosted happiness for up to six months.

The happiness of the groups doing these two exercises improved from each assessment to the next, with their happiness peaking six months after the exercise.

- The "Gratitude Visit" exercise had the biggest immediate effect on happiness and depression; its happiness boost lasted an entire month.
- All the volunteers, *including* those in the placebo group, were happier right after they finished their exercise than before they started it.

It just goes to show that thinking positive really does work. Take time to reflect on the good things in your life, and your happiness will soar.

GREAT-DAY GUIDELINES

Need practice to think positive? Here's a cheat sheet. At first, run down the list when you need to. With time and practice, these behaviors will become second nature—and so will feeling positive and energized.

- Laugh.
- Help someone.
- Monitor your self-talk. Change negative thoughts into positive ones, lose loaded words like *always, never,* and *should,* and use thought-stopping as needed.
- Count your blessings. You can do it in your head or, to enforce the practice, on paper.
- Blast out of your rut. Try something new when you have the chance. You have more chances than you think!
- Face your fear of failure. Run through a situation you fear in your head. Visualize yourself falling on your face—and then getting up.

- Don't dwell in the past or in the future. Learn to live in the moment.
- Cut back on TV. Don't leave it on for "company," either. Try music or public radio instead.
- Identify your personal strengths. Use one in a new way every day for a week.
- Every day, do one thing you have to do, and one thing you want to do.

CHAPTER 6

Recharge with People Power

Did you ever have an absolutely awful day—the kind that goes wrong from the minute you open your eyes in the morning—and have it salvaged by one person? Maybe you talked (or cried) it out with your partner, sister, or best friend. Perhaps, when you hit the gym, the woman on the treadmill next to you struck up a conversation and pulled you out of your funk. Maybe you checked your inbox and found a surprise e-mail from an old friend. Or perhaps it was you who offered a kind word or deed, even though you didn't much want to— you gave blood, or waved a car into the parking space that was rightfully yours.

Whatever the situation, someone touched your heart, or you touched theirs. You felt like you had a place and a purpose in the world, that you were valued and understood, that you *mattered*. This connection, as refreshing as an ice-cold drink on an August afternoon, helped turn your awful day around.

You don't have to be a people person to need people. As social animals, we need others to confide in, share with, chase away our loneliness—and we'll go to great lengths to get the companionship we crave. (Remember Wilson the volleyball in the movie *Castaway*?)

For me, family is the first and strongest bond. I grew up in a large, happy family of five kids—I have three sisters and one brother—and they mean everything to me. Every Sunday we'd go to my grandma's for a big lunch after church. (Mass was a must!) We traded laughter and love, pep talks and advice. Although both my mom and dad have passed, I'm still very close to my brother and sisters. Along with my own family and my best girlfriends, they're part of my life. I don't know what I would do without them!

While family and friends are essential connections, other types are important, too. For example, when you feel a strong bond with your church, a cause, or your community, you feel a part of something larger than yourself. This strong bond not only keeps you going, but very often powers your life.

Here's a simple way to understand the energizing power of connection. Imagine you leave your car headlights on overnight. In the morning, the engine won't turn over—your battery's dead. Your neighbor comes to your rescue and, with jumper cables, connects his car's battery to yours. This jump start from his battery gets your car running again, so its battery can recharge.

A jump start is simply one battery borrowing energy from another. Well, people are like car batteries, too, and our energy works like those jumper cables. Sometimes we're the dead batteries that need a jump start—other people's energy—to recharge. Other times, we use our energy to jump-start someone whose energy has drained away.

If you've ever attended an awesome rock concert, heard a great liturgy in church, or seen a charismatic public speaker in action, you know how you feel afterward: energized and alive. You've experienced the power of connection in action—on a large scale, of course. But it's just as powerful, and more personal, on the smaller stage of everyday life.

All people have a vast amount of untapped energy within them: love! When you're around people who love and value you, you soak up their positivity like a sponge. Your heart opens, and your energy soars. Suddenly you feel on top of the world! In fact, there's even evidence that connecting may improve your immune system. When researchers monitored 276 people between the ages of eighteen and fifty-five, they found that those who had six or more connections were *four times* better at fighting off the viruses that cause colds. At some point, overflowing with positive energy, you give some away. Maybe you make your moody teen his favorite meal, just to show that you love him. Or sign up for the walk against diabetes, organize a lunch for your overworked colleagues to lift their spirits, or knock on an elderly neighbor's door to say hello.

These simple gestures are connection at its best. They touch hearts and give weary souls a shot of positive energy. They feel good, you feel good—that's energy!

Now, I'm not saying you should run yourself ragged. We're all busy, and we all need alone time to "refill the well." But if we're not careful, our busyness can leave us feeling disconnected and alone. Fortunately, there's a cure: Do a kindness for someone else, without expecting anything in return.

At this moment, you possess an awesome power: the power to change the course of another person's day, or even their life, by reaching out. Think back to your last kind word or good deed, when you sought to love rather than be loved, understand rather than be understood, or to comfort rather than be comforted. (That's from one of my favorite prayers, the Prayer of Saint Francis of Assisi.) It felt good, didn't it? That positivity is a

hidden spring of energy, for both you and the person you connect with.

This chapter suggests different ways to connect with both your
family and the friends you do have, as well as the world outside
them. Reach out—you'll feel your energy soar!

HONOR FAMILY TRADITIONS,
OR START NEW ONES

Every year during Thanksgiving week, my family and I head
to the West Coast to see our families. Between Jeff's family
and my own, there are thirty-two of us—our kids have lots of
cousins! We also get together in California for a month in the
summer—we rent a huge beach house and swim, play tennis,
have barbecues, and play volleyball on the beach and backgam-
mon at night. It's my way to keep our two families close. It's
also my joy! My kids have lots of happy memories—"Do you
remember when..."

Now, this doesn't happen by accident—we make it happen!
But all the effort is worth it, because we have so many happy
memories. Handed down from one generation to the next, family
traditions promote closeness, strengthen family bonds, and create
fond memories. If your family doesn't have any traditions, create
new ones.

Before you start a new tradition, think about what you hope to
accomplish. Do you want to bring your family together on a daily
basis, or does a weekly tradition work best for your busy group?
Which holiday does your family particularly enjoy? Do you have
any family traditions now that could use a makeover? One thing
to keep in mind: The best traditions are often the simplest. Don't
go overboard—pick one or two, and make them meaningful.

Use the list of ideas below as a starting point, and tailor them to your family's preferences and circumstances.

Daily Traditions

- Share a kiss and an "I love you" before you leave in the morning.
- Eat dinner together.
- Create a family time when you all stay in the same room.

Weekly Traditions

- Take a Sunday stroll or attend church together.
- Have a midweek pizza-and-movie night.
- Cook Saturday or Sunday breakfast as a family.
- Visit a relative in a retirement or nursing home.

Monthly Traditions

- Have a standing "date" with each child.
- Meet your parents for dinner, or cook them dinner.

Seasonal Traditions

- Plant a garden each spring.
- Pick apples each fall.
- Celebrate the start of summer with a park picnic, or break out a blanket and watch the stars.
- Make a snowman to celebrate the first snow.

Holiday Traditions

- Designate a silly "birthday hat," to be worn at a birthday breakfast or dinner.
- Each Mother's or Father's Day, take a photo with your kids.
- Each Valentine's Day, make one another cards.

- Make a King's Cake together for Fat Tuesday.
- Each St. Patrick's Day, serve a different green food for dinner.

Christmas Traditions
- Go to a tree farm and cut your own tree.
- Put a new ornament on the tree each year.
- Have a neighborhood open house.
- Give everyone silly new pajamas on Christmas Eve.

MAKE TIME FOR THOSE YOU LOVE

If you're married with children, like me, and have a large circle of friends, the problem may not be getting connected, but staying that way. We're all so busy that you may find that, despite your best intentions, you really aren't sharing quality time with the people you care most about. A broken lunch date with a girlfriend, a school play you didn't make it to, a postponed date night...these missed opportunities add up, until one day you find yourself missing a person who lives in your own house! Here's how to build stronger connections with the people in your life that you care about most:

- **Schedule "together time."** This is a biggie for me! My husband is a very busy sports attorney, and between filming my TV shows, public appearances, and book tours, I'm constantly on the go, too. But just when you're the busiest, make an ironclad commitment to making the time. Put down this book and set a date right now, whether for a movie or a night out to dinner with another couple, while you're thinking of it!
- **Start a monthly girls' night out.** Once a month, I get together with a special group of women: the mothers of the girls who played lacrosse with my girls. These young women were teammates for more than ten years, and all of us moms had been on the sidelines together, cheering them on. Our

girls are all at different colleges now, but we moms still get together once a month to reminisce. It's just this wonderful bond we share.

Do you have a tight-knit group of friends you almost never see? Go on…call those BFFs and pick a date, a time, and a place! The talk, laughter, and camaraderie will ease your stress and do your heart good. Pick a restaurant one of you has heard about, go to a movie together, or just hang out at home. You'll have fun and make memories that will last a lifetime!

- **Exercise together.** About five years ago, a group of my girlfriends and I started a fun way to stay close: "birthday walks." On our birthdays, we go to the birthday girl's house and walk in her neighborhood, followed by a special birthday breakfast or lunch. Those walks are our gifts to one another, and we get our thirty minutes of exercise in—together. It's so much fun—we catch up, share some laughter, and then go our separate ways, refreshed.

  Could you make a standing date to walk with your best friend in your neighborhood or hers? Or ask your partner to work out with you, so you can motivate and encourage each other? If you have kids, make exercise a family affair—join a gym with a pool, or take a Spinning class together. You could also walk the dog, take a hike, or ride bikes around the park—all of these activities give you the chance to catch up as you get fit.

CONNECT WITH AN OLD FRIEND

Every few months, I call my best girlfriend from college, Maryjane, just to catch up. I've done this for twenty years, and our friendship is still going strong. It feels so good to talk to, or hear from, an old friend who has known you all your life!

Old friends are special because they're a living bridge to your past. They knew you, and maybe your family, while you were growing up, and have memories of you that no one else does (including stories you'll take to your grave with you!). In a way, when you reconnect with these friends, you reconnect with yourself. So pick up the phone—you're bound to find that the years melt away. Tease each other about nerdy prom dates. Giggle over the crazy stunts you pulled. Play the "where are they now" game with mutual acquaintances. The glow from one heartfelt gabfest can rev you up for days!

If you haven't been in touch for years, you may be hesitant to call out of the blue. Test the waters first—find a friend on Facebook and write on her personal page. Or if you know where she lives, pop a card in the mail, along with a photo from the old days.

Speaking of photos, photo sharing is a great way to keep the connection open—you can share photos from the old days as well as those of your kids. There are many photo-sharing sites that offer an easy way to share pictures. Just sign up, download pictures to create an album, name your album, and e-mail the link to your friend.

PEACE POCKET

Daydream at a Window

Fix yourself a cup of tea, cozy up to a big picture window, and drink in the world that surrounds you. People watch, or appreciate the birds within view and the clouds floating by.

PLAN A REUNION

You may see your parents every day (I wish I could!), but when was the last time you saw Aunt Betty or Uncle Pete, or the cousins you visited every summer when you were a kid?

Family is like a garden: You have to cultivate it. But when you do, the rewards are great. Reconnecting with or meeting family members who live in different parts of the country can solidify your family bonds and bring back happy memories. My mother's sisters, my aunt Loretta and aunt Mary, live in Lockport, New York. We fly them in for special family events—graduations, weddings, our weeklong family get-togethers. They love seeing family, and I love to see them—they remind me so much of my mom. Family reunions can also be rewarding for your children, who get to see their family tree up close.

Of course, there are other types of reunions. You might reconnect with your BFFs from college, high school, or even grade school, or catch up with the friends you made while in the military. One type of reunion—for co-workers—has become quite popular, especially among those who worked at a company that no longer exists. When you share work gripes and triumphs with a group of people for years, those in the group become like family (even

REVIVE IN 5!

Take a Walk Down Memory Lane

Whenever my sisters and I get together, one of us ends up pulling out the family albums. We spend hours talking about the good times and trading memories of Mom and Dad. Why not relive your own precious memories with your best friend, parent, sibling, or partner? It's a wonderful way to spend meaningful time together. Dig out your old photo albums, scrapbooks, wedding album, baby books, or home movies and laugh at the fashions and hairstyles. This is a fabulous way to relive funny moments, share stories others may have forgotten, or honor a beloved relative who has passed away.

the grumpy-but-lovable ones!), and you miss them when you no longer see them every day.

While it can be a challenge to plan a reunion, it can also be fun, and many websites offer step-by-step guidance, including how to pick a location, get the word out, and keep costs down. Most of these sites are devoted to family reunions, but some also offer help with other types.

TURN YOUR WORKPLACE INTO A COMMUNITY

Where do you spend the majority of your week? What stresses you out more than anything? Work, of course! Nothing can reduce workplace gloom and tension as well as a spirit of we're-all-in-it-together camaraderie. No matter how gloomy and silent the atmosphere, one person—you—can turn it around. Take the reins and make it happen!

Fit your plan to the realities of your workplace, and think about where your officemates would be most likely to gather. If you don't have a break room or cafeteria, maybe you send out a group e-mail: "Next Friday is the first monthly Friday-afternoon lunch at the local pizza joint. RSVP." Even if only three others accept, it's a start—and after a few months of pizza and conversation, no one will want to be left out! (If you're on a diet, factor a slice or two into that day's meal plan.) Or arrange a "fitness Friday"—a quick walk and lunch afterward. My girlfriends and I do this a lot, but it would be a perfect way to connect with co-workers, too.

You could also see if there's interest in forming a workplace bowling league—include your co-workers' partners, too. Knocking over pins on Tuesday can make everyone's Wednesday more productive and engender a spirit of cooperation that lingers straight through till Friday.

GET TO KNOW YOUR NEIGHBORS

I love mine—we have so much fun! After a blizzard a year or so back, we all spent hours in thigh-deep snow, shoveling ourselves out. For four days straight, we shouted encouragement and threw a few friendly snowballs as we shoveled, then ended up at one neighbor's house or another for an early dinner or a glass of wine.

If you don't know your neighbors, reach out. Chances are, several are just as eager to make new friends as you are. The next time you and a neighbor are taking out the trash or walking to the mailbox at the same time, smile and exchange a few words. Repeat with the lady across the street, or the older woman who lives downstairs from you. After a month of that, take it up a notch. One afternoon, as you chat over the fence, or by the mailbox, invite one neighbor, then another, over for a quick cup of coffee or tea.

Reach out to new neighbors, too. For ten years now, my girls and I have welcomed every new neighbor with a loaf of my home-made pumpkin bread and insider information on their new neighborhood (like which place has the best pizza). It feels good to help, and I've ended up with a circle of very close neighbors who are always there to help.

RENEW YOUR FAITH, OR JUST GET SPIRITUAL

This is another biggie for me. My faith is important to me, and I'd hope my girls feel the same way. That's why, as much as we can, we attend church together as a family. I love when a priest gives a wonderful sermon...sometimes I cry, I get so inspired and emotional!

Even if you don't practice a particular faith, consider that spirituality can help you live your life with positive energy, and connect you to a power greater than yourself. If you grew up in a specific faith but no longer attend services, consider giving your church another try. If you're spiritual but not religious, you might attend a nondenominational church, or "sample" several different faiths. Just sitting in church for an hour a week can make you feel good, particularly if the church has a choir. Gospel churches often have wonderful choirs, and the energy they generate is electrifying!

VOLUNTEER, FAMILY-STYLE

While it might be a challenge to coordinate everyone's schedules, volunteering as a family has many worthwhile benefits. Your children watch everything you do—if you give back to the community, you show them firsthand how good it feels to help others and enact positive change. It's also a valuable way for you to get to know organizations in the community and find resources and activities for your children and family.

REVIVE IN 5!

5 Easy Ways to Plug into People Power

1. Pack food for your local food bank.
2. Hang out with your pooch at the local dog park.
3. Walk or bike to support a cause.
4. Volunteer to usher at your community theater.
5. Attend a town or city council meeting.

WHEN YOU'RE TOO CONNECTED

As energizing and life affirming as strong personal connections are, there can be too much of a good thing. If you sing in the church choir, mentor an underprivileged teen in your community, coach your child's soccer team, *and* run the neighborhood watch association, maybe your main energy problem isn't too few connections, but too many!

We'll cover this in more depth in the next chapter, but if you have too many obligations and not enough time to catch your breath, it's time to say those three little words: "Sorry, I can't." Saying no doesn't make you selfish. It makes you honest. It means that you know your limits. Spend your energy on the commitments you already have, and remember to save some for yourself, too!

5 Ways to Connect in 12 Minutes or Less

To show you how simple it can be to forge stronger bonds, I've listed five ways to connect in twelve minutes or less. Try one or more of them today.

1. **Support local shops.** Quick—name your favorite restaurant, café, or shop. Did you choose a local business, or a national chain? While chain restaurants and big-box stores are convenient and offer competitive prices, they can't match the "flavor" of small, unique shops with local character. A quick way to connect with your community is to shop at local businesses as much as you can. For example, buy local fruit and veggies at the weekly farmer's market, pick up bread at the local bakery rather than at the convenience store, and sip a cappuccino at a local bookstore at least as often as you frequent the national chains. Also, before you drive to a big-box store, consider whether you can find the same item at a local business, which depends on your patronage to survive. When you support locally owned businesses, you help maintain your community's distinctive flavor and rub elbows with your neighbors. You're also likely to receive top-notch customer service. Once they know you, they'll treat you like family!

2. **Write a thank-you note.** My mother made us kids write out our thanks for every birthday and Christmas gift, and I'll bet yours did, too. Sadly, writing a thank-you note is a vanishing art,

but I still make my girls do it. (It's not easy, but I try!) In this age of e-mails, Tweets, and Facebook updates, a handwritten note on lovely paper says, *You're special.* But don't only write notes for gifts wrapped in paper. Think of a recipient who gave you the most special gift of all: a thoughtful word or act, either recently or in the past.

Buy some nice stationery or tasteful note cards. Your words don't have to be polished, just sincere. Your neighbor trimmed your hedges along with theirs? Surely that deserves a thank-you. Did your uncle loan you the down payment for your first car years ago? Tell him you still remember the kindness. There's no shortage of people who've touched your life in some way. Maybe you'd like to thank your hairstylist for the first haircut in years that makes you feel pretty or sexy, or your parents for standing by you during a difficult time. You'll feel as good writing your note as they'll feel reading it—and unlike an e-mail, it will be saved and treasured.

3. **Look in on an older neighbor.** Many elderly men and women live alone—their spouses and friends have passed on, and their children may live far away. Drop by to introduce yourself and offer a helping hand. Once or twice a week, see how they're doing and offer to pick up any supplies, including prescriptions, they may need. Send your teen out to shovel their walkway after a snowstorm. If you're going to the mall, offer them a ride. You'll feel good that you've touched someone's life. Plus, older people are often an amazing untapped source of knowledge and wisdom. You may end up with a true friend who adds immeasurably to your life.

4. **Pick it up even if you didn't drop it.** When you walk through parks or other public places and see litter, pick it up and throw it in a nearby trash can. This small gesture says so much. Because

you've made that public space more pleasant for the next people who use it, your gesture says that you value your community, and that you believe that we're all responsible for making our little piece of the world a nicer place to live. Plus, if someone witnesses your good deed, they may be inspired to do the same!

5. **Treat strangers to small social graces.** When I get into an elevator, I always smile and make eye contact. If this little gesture gives even one of my fellow elevator riders a tiny mood boost, that smile was well worth it! Try it the next time you board an elevator. You might also wave at neighbors you know by sight but haven't met (and then make a point to introduce yourself), exchange pleasantries with the teller at the bank, or ask a co-worker you don't know well about his or her recent vacation. When you employ these social graces, you set an example for others, who may be inspired to follow your lead.

ENERGY MAKEOVER!

AMY TRANSUE, 52
HOMETOWN: SCHNECKSVILLE, PENNSYLVANIA
OCCUPATION: STAY-AT-HOME MOM

Amy Transue is a wife and stay-at-home mom of six children in their teens and twenties—one married, one away at college, and four still at home, two of whom she homeschools. "I love my family, but find that my energy to keep up with them is diminishing," says Amy. Amy's eighty-one-year-old mother recently moved in with her family, adding to her caregiving responsibilities.

Her schedule is frantic, Amy explains. "From the time I get up, I hit the ground running—supervising breakfast for everyone,

exercise, however, you may be experiencing a common symptom of perimenopause. In fact, it's *very* common—I have the same experience at night sometimes myself. The day after "one of those nights," catch a twenty-minute catnap while your homeschoolers do independent work. (Give them a study hall or reading period!)

Strength training is important, too—it will tone your muscles and power up your energy. You can do it at home, and all you'll need is a few sets of weights that you can pick up at any big-box store. You'll find your twenty-minute shape-up energy workout in chapter 12. I guarantee these energy-boosting moves will firm your muscles and keep your stamina high!

CHAPTER 7

A Balanced Life Is an Energized Life

Balance? Tell me about it! Achieving a balance between work and family is as tough for me as it probably is for you. The most important things in my life are my family, my friends, and my faith. I never want to miss one of my daughters' lacrosse games, a girlfriend's birthday party, a Saturday-night dinner with my husband, or family time on Sunday. My career is also important to me—knowing that I'm out there helping people get fit and live well gives my life joy and purpose.

Family, faith, work, close relationships—as you can see, I have a lot on my plate. Although I can't do it all, I sure try! So I *always* struggle with balance. It's not easy to fly across the country on business, leaving my family behind. It's also not easy to pass on a project because it would take me away from my family for too long, or juggle multiple family or work obligations because I need a girls' night out!

While it's hard to be pulled in so many directions, I've learned through the years how to achieve the fine art of balance (most of the time). Although it's not always easy to attain, I strive for it, because it's the key to living the happy, healthy life I want—and that I want for you, too!

The key to balance? In a word: *priorities*. To find balance, you decide what in life is most important to you—your priorities. Then you put those things first. Simple to say, hard to do…but it *can* be done, if you want it badly enough.

I hope you do, because the benefits are huge. For one thing, you save your physical, mental, and emotional energy for those all-important priorities, and the extraneous things that used to pull you in a thousand different directions fall by the wayside. For another thing, when you live in balance, you tend to live your values, and that always feels great!

Is balancing ever easy? Absolutely not! Balanced women don't "do it all," and Superwoman exists only in the movies. I figure if I can put my family to bed happy, get a good night's sleep, keep everyone in clean (if wrinkled) clothing, and get in my daily thirty-minute workout, I'm doing great!

In the end, balance means that you accomplish your "must-dos," like work, with a positive attitude, but live for your "want-to-dos"—family, hobbies, worship, fun. You know what your priorities are and can juggle them like a champ. You're challenged by your life, but relaxed enough to enjoy it.

In this chapter, I'll share my strategies for a balanced life. Here's a sneak preview:

DENISE'S FORMULA FOR A BALANCED LIFE
Be flexible.
Accept a less-than-tidy home.
Learn to manage your time.
Ask for help.
No! (Just say it—it's okay!)
Carve out family and "me" time.
Enjoy life!

Living in balance is a journey, not a destination. Armed with your priorities, you decide what's important to you, recognize your power to make choices, do what you can, and leave the rest. Above all, don't measure balance by how many to-dos you cross off your list, but by how much you enjoy your life!

In this chapter, I'll explain how this concept works for me in my life, and how it can work for you, too. Now, this formula isn't foolproof—you can't, and shouldn't, try to follow every strategy perfectly. (Perfectionism has no place in a balanced life.) The balanced life tips in the sections below are guidelines. Follow them as best you can each day, and know that's enough.

Get ready to find the balance that works for you. When you do, it won't take long for your energy to soar!

BE FLEXIBLE

There's a reason someone (most likely a woman) invented the schedule and the to-do list: They make life more predictable, and therefore more in our control. The kids leave for school weekday mornings at seven thirty and you tackle your household chores; you put the baby down for a nap every afternoon after lunch; you take your daily walk promptly before or after work. When you do the same things at the same time, life runs more smoothly. In theory, anyway!

But then that schedule comes apart, and that list might as well be written in the sand at low tide. Your kids miss the bus. Your computer seizes up, and you lose your report that's due the next day. You have a party planned, or a meeting to attend...and your child comes down with an ear infection.

A balanced life is one that allows, even expects, a bit of chaos. The antidote: flexibility! When you go with the flow, rather than try to bend life to your will, you conserve energy (and preserve your sanity!). Life is unpredictable. Stuff happens! Accept it, and roll with the punches; you'll be less likely to feel stressed or upset, which expends precious emotional or mental energy.

There's an old story that illustrates the importance of flexibility.

The morning after a terrible storm, a farmer and his son walked their property to see if the weather had caused any damage. As they drew closer to their small stream, they saw that the high winds had uprooted their huge old oak. But the graceful old willow

---

REVIVE IN 5!

Plan for More Energy!

Sundays in my house can start out nuts—my family has tons of commitments, from church to sports to get-togethers. But the day always ends in a spirit of calm, as everyone winds down from an active weekend and mentally preps for another hectic week. One thing I do, without fail, is jot down my list of must-dos. It takes just five minutes, but it can save me precious hours of time and a lot of energy.

This coming Sunday night, take a minute or two to assess what you need to do in the coming week—appointments, meetings to attend, exams to study for. Then write them all down! Why not treat yourself to a pretty planner or notebook that slips easily into your purse for this very purpose?

In the list, be sure to pencil in quality time for yourself and your family as well as your must-dos. Actually, write that family or personal time in pen—it's that non-negotiable! When you make the time to connect with family and friends, you add balance to your life and also recharge your mental and emotional batteries, which will make you more efficient in the long run. *You don't have to do everything; just do what really matters!*

near the stream, its thin, frail branches stirring gently in the breeze, had weathered the storm just fine.

The boy wondered why the thick, strong oak had been destroyed, while a weak willow was still standing. The father replied, "The oak tree fell because it could not bend in the wind. But the willow was able to bend, so the storm couldn't bring it down."

The moral of the story: Bend with the wind, and you will never break!

Now, there are times when you absolutely cannot achieve balance. For example, you may experience a family or work crisis that requires your undivided attention and energy. That's where perspective comes in. Perspective is a kind of mental balance—it's the time-honored *This, too, shall pass* approach. When things get totally crazy, do what you need to do to weather that storm. Then, when life gets back to normal, take the time to refresh and rejuvenate!

ACCEPT A LESS-THAN-TIDY HOME

Although I am lucky to have a housekeeper two mornings a week to do the hard-core cleaning, there are still five other days where the housework is all up to me—cleaning, grocery shopping, errands, the whole deal. Believe me, my home is far from perfect. My daughters' rooms have piles of clothes on the floor, my desk overflows with bills and paperwork, and our family room often looks, well, lived in. (Thank God I have a tidy husband!) And yet my family is happy in our not-always-immaculate home.

I'm not saying that you should turn a blind eye to housework, especially if you're a person who simply cannot function in mess and clutter. But seek balance between keeping a home that could be photographed for a magazine, and a comfortably lived-in look.

Ask yourself: If your Christmas decorations stay up a week or two too long, will the world come to an end? Balance is achieved over time, not all at one moment in time, and not in every part of your life at once.

In order to balance your busy life, you need to know what you value and what you hope to achieve, and then prioritize. If an immaculate home is important to you, go for it. But remember, if you're frantically busy, something's got to give, and better a pile of laundry in the hallway than an unhappy family or an unhappy you! Pick your battles, and in times of conflict or indecisiveness, ask yourself what truly matters. Chances are, it won't be that the stovetop needs to be scrubbed!

Do what needs to be done and let the rest go. It's also helpful to break cleaning into chunks, rather than tackle it all on weekends, which cuts into family or that all-important time to yourself.

What I like to do is pop in one of my favorite CDs and clean for ten or fifteen minutes—as opposed to an hour or more. I focus on just one room, too—for me, it's my kitchen, for you it might be your family room. Talk about a shot of energy—the music brightens my mood, and I feel like I've accomplished something! One other thing I do is, no matter what, empty the sink, wash dirty dishes, and wipe it all down before I head off to bed. Walking into the kitchen for a cup of coffee, only to be greeted by a stack of dirty dishes, is a major energy drainer!

Go for the Goals!

Where do you want to be in three weeks? Three months? A year? In five years? Have you thought about it? If not, it may be time to think about what you want to achieve in your life and set some goals!

Setting goals motivates you—in other words, it focuses your energy. Setting goals, and then achieving them, can also help balance your life, because the goals you set will reflect your priorities.

You'll want to set two types of goals: short-term and long-term.

Short-term goals are those that you can realize in the near future, such as in a day, within the week, or even in a few months. Examples of short-term goals include finishing a project at work or getting your shopping for the holidays done.

Long-term goals are those you plan to achieve over a year or more. Because it takes a while to achieve them, they usually are meaningful and give you a sense of greater purpose. An example of a long-term goal is finally starting the home-based business of your dreams.

At any given time, try to have at least one short-term and one long-term goal. Having short-term goals provides you with a sense of accomplishment as you wait to achieve your long-term goals. Similarly, having a long-term goal gives your life a sense of meaning and purpose.

Before you set your goals, take a few moments to list the things that matter most to you—your priorities. That requires honesty and thought. Once you identify them, structure your goals around them.

Set your long-term goals first—this will give you a sense of direction and purpose. Then choose one or more short-term goals you need to accomplish to reach your long-term goal, the stepping-stones that bring you along the path toward your long-term goals. By setting and focusing on these short-term goals and realizing them, you build momentum toward achieving your long-term plans.

For example, if you have a long-term goal of learning to speak French, your short-term goals may include getting a language-learning CD out of the library to listen to on your commute each morning,

signing up for and taking a class, or finding a native speaker to practice your conversation. Maybe you'll even want to start saving so
you can reward yourself with a trip to Paris to celebrate when you
achieve your goal!

Right now, write down one long-term and one short-term goal.
Include how you will achieve it, along with a deadline. For example,
one of my short-term goals is to get to every one of both of my
daughters' lacrosse games. I won't travel when they have games, and
I work my schedule around them. So far, I've made 90 percent of them
this season, and that gives me great pride! My long-term goal is to stay
fit and healthy forever, and I work a little on that each and every day!

PEACE POCKET

Listen to a Relaxation CD

Invest in one or more CDs that offer sounds that soothe you—
birds, waves, gentle rain. Close your eyes, do some deep breathing,
and soak up these peaceful sounds.

LEARN TO MANAGE YOUR TIME

In my life, the race is on from the moment I open my eyes in the
morning until my head hits the pillow! I couldn't do it all if I
hadn't learned, over the years, how to manage my time effectively.
It isn't a mysterious concept—it's simply a way to find the time
for all the things you want and need to do. Knowing your priorities and goals in life is a huge part of time management, too. That
ensures that you use your most precious commodity—time—more
wisely.

There are many, many great books on time management that
will help you organize your schedule so that you have more time

than you thought to live a happy, balanced life. But a few basic principles can help right now: Prioritize your tasks, and control procrastination.

To prioritize tasks, make a list of all your must-dos for the day. Then rate these tasks by how important or urgent they are.

Let Go of Perfectionism!

Perfectionism has no place in a balanced life, because it sucks up time and energy that you could use in other areas of your life. Here are a few tips for controlling the urge to do everything perfectly all the time:

- **Be realistic!** Know the difference between reasonable goals and those that are impossible to achieve. Example: A reasonable goal for a working mom is to clean the house from top to bottom once every two weeks. Clean it every day? Not so much! When you set reasonable goals, you'll feel great when you achieve them, rather than shame and guilt when you don't.

- **Talk yourself out of the fiddles.** Do you spend time fiddling with details that only you will notice (for example, scrubbing the corners of the bathroom with a toothbrush, or folding clothing just so?), then scramble to finish the rest of the day's work? If so, you're frittering away precious mental energy! The next time you're tempted to "fiddle," come up with a mantra that brings fresh perspective to a stuck situation. For example, "That'll do for now," or "It's good enough."

- **Enjoy the journey!** As you move toward your goal, enjoy the process, rather than living only for the end result. That way, you get to live life as it unfolds. Perfectionism takes the spontaneity out of life. Remember to be kind to yourself, and do the best you can!

Urgent tasks must be dealt with immediately to avoid a problem, while *important* tasks are those that are meaningful to you, such as time with your family, your daily walk, or volunteer work at your church.

On my list, urgent tasks might include taking the car into the shop or going grocery shopping. Important tasks might include getting in my workout, helping one of my daughters with a school paper or other project, and planning one of our annual family get-togethers (my favorite thing to do!).

After you've rated the items on your list, scrutinize it. Is there a task on your list that, on second thought, isn't urgent after all? Can you think of any ways you could redirect your time to activities that reflect your priorities in life?

Time management also means controlling procrastination. Use a day planner or notebook to plan your day or week. Just seeing on paper that there is a time to get your tasks done can help you get to work.

Another helpful tip: Break up large tasks. For example, if you haven't started a paper that you know will take you two weeks to finish, break up your work into one-hour blocks over fourteen days. It's easier to face an unpleasant task if you know you don't have to spend more than an hour at a time on it!

ASK FOR HELP!

As women, we take on the world—and *our* worlds—every day. We're the primary caretakers of our marriages and kids. Whether or not we work outside the home, we're the main cooks, nannies, laundry ladies, errand runners, and chauffeurs, all rolled into one. Oh, and let's not forget our duties as personal shoppers, accountants, and all-around cheerleaders and enforcers. We wear a heck of a lot of hats! In fact, it's been estimated that if the average homemaker drew a salary, her labor would be worth $30,000 a year!

I am extremely lucky. Jeff couldn't be more supportive, and he and the girls regularly pitch in to help around the house when I just can't do it all myself. But you know what? Sometimes I have to ask—and I feel just fine about that!

Do you ask for help when you need it? I admit, I had to learn to do it myself. When my first, Kelly, was born, I tried to do it all—take care of a newborn as well as do all the shopping, cooking, and cleaning on my own. Well, I ran myself ragged—and by the time she was six weeks old, I broke down and asked for help. I remember my girlfriends would come over and watch Kelly for me so I could run to the grocery store without an infant.

Everyone needs a hand once in a while, even you! When you ask for help, you show that you care about and value yourself, and have enough self-confidence to *allow* others to help you. By delegating, you add balance to your life, and take care of *you*. You also conserve valuable energy that can be used elsewhere, either to care for others or for yourself. When you share your to-do list, you create an opportunity to deepen your relationships with your family, employer, or others. After all, being part of a family, workplace, or community is about give and take. Equalize that equation—give others the chance to give to you!

Think about the way you ask for help. Do you bark out orders and get frustrated when they're not carried out? Next time ask with a smile and a positive attitude, and have a plan in mind.

For example, tell your family what you've planned for the weekend—say, both yard work and a get-together with friends. Then let them help you plan. Give them each a job to do, and check in during the week to assess their progress. Or share with your neighbor, who also has a school-aged child, about your volunteer work with the school raffle, and ask if she might lend a hand.

Take off one or more of those hats—you don't have to wear all of them at the same time. When you delegate, the downtime you gain will revive and restore you. You'll be more efficient, yes, but also happier and more energetic. The next time you're in meltdown mode, take a deep breath and say those three little words: "Can you help?" They're some of the most energizing words in the English language!

NO! (JUST SAY IT—IT'S OKAY!)

Does your to-do list make you want to run and hide? Mine does sometimes, particularly because I always have several projects I'm working on and my husband and daughters are also involved in plenty of activities and events.

I find that it's helpful to decide which obligations in my life are the most important—then I can prioritize. As for the others, I can't do it all, and I sometimes have to say a polite but firm no. For example, I've recently had to say no to certain jobs because they take me away from my family for too long. (But I always try to go the extra mile for family and friends, because *they* are my priorities!)

Saying no protects your time and energy, but it can be hard to muster the courage to do it—especially if you're someone who likes to please others. To get into practice, try saying, "No, but thank you for thinking of me." It's gracious to thank people for an opportunity when you turn them down, and you'll be less likely to feel guilty afterward. You can also give a reason you can't help, if you have one and are comfortable sharing the information. If you don't have a specific reason you want to share, you can just say that you've been overextending yourself lately and need to cut back.

Yes, you'll feel guilty for a few minutes, but think how relieved you'll be afterward! I believe that it's possible to pitch in and help your friends and neighbors and kids without feeling overwhelmed and overcommitted—just decide which efforts you want to make and don't be afraid to turn down the rest. You owe it to yourself!

And once you've learned to say no to others, it's time to start saying yes to you! Read on to find out what I mean.

CARVE OUT FAMILY AND PERSONAL TIME

Jeff and I grew up knowing the comfort and security of strong family bonds, and no matter how hectic our lives get, we always fit in family time. (The messiness of our family room proves it!) We each also manage to squeeze in a bit of time out with our friends—Jeff plays tennis with his buddies, while I go for a walk with my girlfriends.

How about you? No time for either your family or yourself, you say? Well, a balanced life isn't about "getting it all done." It's about knowing what's important in your life, and giving it top priority. It's about turning off your cell phone and e-mail and bonding with the people you share your bathroom with!

Think of it this way. Would you skip out on work, a parent–teacher conference, or a doctor's appointment? Of course not! Well, your time with your family and friends—and yourself—deserves the same commitment. Just as an apple a day keeps the doctor away, regular "dates" with your family, your friends, or yourself add balance to your busy schedule.

Make sure to ink in family time as a non-negotiable part of your schedule—the rewards of a strong family are enormous and last a lifetime. An easy way to do that is to play together as a family—play board games or Frisbee, ride bikes or hike together, or simply watch a movie together. Enjoying these activities as a family helps build and strengthen family bonds and establishes memories in the making. It also lets your children know that their family actually likes spending time with them. What a confidence booster!

Guard this personal time passionately, and don't let work or other distractions intrude. Stop checking e-mail and cell phones so often. Very few of us are so important that we need our phones on 24/7!

Turn Off the Gadgets!

I love my cell phone, I really do. I can send pictures on it, I can get urgent e-mails on it, and, of course, I can keep in touch with family and friends no matter where I am. But sometimes, I just need to turn that sucker off for an hour or two to get dinner going or simply sit in my backyard and enjoy the sunshine and fresh air. Turning off my cell phone is one way I achieve balance between work and play. When I turn it off, I cease to be a human *doing*, and start feeling like a human *being* again!

BlackBerries, pagers, e-mail...today's electronic gadgets are a great way to stay connected to family and friends far away. But these devices can be double-edged swords, too. When you feel that you have to be available to your employer 24/7, the line between home and work blurs. In fact, there is no line between the two. Where's the balance in that?

Make a conscious decision to separate your work time from personal time. If you're your own boss, it's up to you to create boundaries that keep work from intruding on family time.

For example, when you're having family time at night, or on the weekends, turn off your cell phone and put away your laptop computer. Don't worry—if it's important, they'll call again!

Schedule time for yourself, too, for exercise, hobbies, or just to relax, refocus, and recharge. When you say yes to taking time for yourself, you are honoring your need to play as well as to work, whether you're a stay-at-home mom or a jet-setting business-woman. No matter if it's dinner with friends, an intense workout at the gym, or a cup of coffee and your favorite magazine, you must have some time for yourself—you've earned it! Honor it just as you would any other must-do in your life.

ENJOY LIFE!

If you often feel as if you're living in fast-forward, trying to stay one step ahead of the craziness we call life, you're not alone—even I feel that way! There's the work project that's due next week, the preparations for the upcoming baby shower or birthday party to attend to, or the study session to help your son or daughter (or grandchild) get ready for a test—but there doesn't seem to be any time for fun. And just when you think you finally have it all under control—here come some more tasks and responsibilities!

It's tough to replenish your energy when you virtually never stop to catch your breath. Time out! The nonstop roller coaster of life might not cut you any slack, but you can give *yourself* a break.

Every day contains an abundance of simple pleasures. (In fact, I'll get to that in the next chapter.) But if you move too fast, you will overlook most of them. It's time to start living for today! If you don't, you're going to turn around one day and wonder what you've been busy with your whole life, and when you get to start enjoying it. We all need to take a step back and let ourselves relax and recharge—and make time for the things that are really important.

What I want you to focus on is investing a little time in the here and now to enjoy yourself. Sit down and read to your child or grandchild, pick up the phone and call that friend you've been meaning to talk to for months now, or just sit by a window and watch the beautiful sunset instead of rushing right by it. All your tasks and responsibilities can be taken care of in due time; you'll see.

Every week, set aside time for an activity that you enjoy, and that you know will rejuvenate you. Let everyone know that that time is yours and can't be rescheduled. Those few hours can be spent working out, getting a manicure, practicing yoga, starting a new hobby—or simply sitting down in a quiet room with a good book or your journal.

Think that's selfish? No way—that's balance! Every woman needs to recharge her batteries, and that's okay! You can afford a daily thirty-minute break to just enjoy yourself. In fact, you can't afford *not* to take it. This half hour will restore your energy so you can hit your to-do list with newfound vigor. Once you get into the habit of spending non-negotiable time with yourself, you'll start to see a difference—in both your energy and your mood!

ENERGY MAKEOVER!

KRISTEN SUNDBY HUTCHINS, 28
HOMETOWN: SACRAMENTO, CALIFORNIA
OCCUPATION: POLICE OFFICER

Kristen Sundby Hutchins's major energy drainer, she wrote me, is double trouble: a frantic schedule, and no personal time. "My current assignment is to help fellow officers manage stress during tough times," she told me. "I work four ten-plus-hour days a week, with Friday through Sunday off. However, I am on call even on my days off." Despite the demands of her job, however, Kristen loves it. "The rewards of helping others are priceless."

Her amazing husband, also a police officer, and her beautiful eleven-year-old daughter are priceless, too, Kristen adds—but her go-go-go lifestyle is wearing her down. She gets up every morning at five and spends a full day caring for others. She gets home at around 6 PM, puts on her wife-and-mom hat, and faces a new round of commitments—fix dinner, do chores, help her daughter with homework and spend quality time with her, and pack her bag for the next day. "By the time I fall into bed with my husband to watch the news, I am exhausted and have done nothing for myself," she writes. "I'd love to read before bed—I buy books constantly, but never read them—but 'news hour' with my husband is our bonding time."

Kristen is asleep by 11 PM, "and only a bomb would wake me!" Sometimes that happens, literally. She routinely gets called in the middle of the night to deal with hostage situations, critical incidents, or troubled officers. Sometimes both Kristen *and* her husband get called in, and they have to call one of their moms to stay with their daughter.

One thing Kristen has going for her: She lives a healthy lifestyle. "As a police officer, I have to stay in shape," she says. "I eat well, but always on the go and occasionally too little." (Kristen is five foot seven and 128 pounds, and estimates that she consumes from fourteen to sixteen hundred calories a day.) She runs regularly and works out, too. That's a good thing, because Kristen and her husband are thinking about having another child. "So I've scaled back the running and am trying to eat more," she writes. "I could sleep more, too—I get between 5.5 and 6.5 hours a night."

Kristen does enjoy some time off, but again, she doesn't get a whole lot of time to herself to relax and decompress. "My husband and I get away occasionally for weekends, as long as someone covers my calls," she writes. "We take vacations, both alone and with our daughter, and my parents sometimes come along." Every spring, they get away to Mendocino, on the Northern California coast, for a weekend. They hike, walk on the beach, and are in bed by eight every night. "It's low-key and calming, and best of all, the phones don't work very well there!"

She is also lucky to have a wonderful support system. Unfortunately, she doesn't see them in person very often. "My parents live minutes away, but I see them maybe two to three times a month. I have good friends, but again, my schedule doesn't permit me to see them much; our contact is primarily through text and e-mail," Kristen writes. "And although my husband encourages me to take time for myself, that doesn't always happen. I try to find balance in my life and care for myself, but after caring for everyone else, sometimes there just isn't time."

Well, Kristen, first the good news. You love your job, have strong, close relationships, and are about to expand your family. You've got a lot going for you! Your high-stress profession makes you a prime candidate for compassion fatigue, however. (You probably already know that!) So you *need* that time to yourself to recharge your emotional and mental energy. Fortunately, I see many opportunities for you to do that—you just need to take them!

First, let's work on energizing your lifestyle. It sounds like you are very health-conscious. At five foot seven and 128 pounds, your body mass index (BMI) puts you in a healthy weight range, and it's great that you're trying to eat more in preparation for pregnancy. However, eating more may do wonders for your energy, too.

An active woman and a runner should consume about two thousand calories a day. Since you eat on the go, or at your desk, stock up on quick-and-healthy options: whole-grain crackers with natural peanut butter and banana, yogurt and cheese sticks, raisins, nuts, smoothies made with skim milk, fresh fruit, and whey protein. Add energizing baked potatoes, beans, or whole-grain pasta to your lunch and dinner menus, along with fish, poultry, or lean meat for protein. If you can, cook for the week on weekends—maybe your husband or daughter can join you in the kitchen!

One last thing: Because you're trying to conceive, be sure to get four hundred micrograms of the B vitamin folic acid every day *before* you get pregnant. This will help prevent birth defects of the brain and spinal cord. (I used to work as an ambassador for the March of Dimes, so preventing spina bifida is important to me.) Take a daily multivitamin with four hundred micrograms of folic acid, and eat foods rich in folate, the natural form of the vitamin, such as spinach, kale, and orange juice.

With an active schedule like yours, and frequent middle-of-the-night wake-ups, sleep is a priority. Could you and your husband turn in when your daughter does, push up your bonding time by an hour, and turn out the lights by 10 PM? At the very least, the day after one of those late nights, shut the door to your office, lower the shades, and catnap for twenty minutes. There's a trade-off, of course—you may have to let the house go a bit. But sleep is more important!

Now for that "me time." You have weekends off. Once a month, get your on-call covered, wave good-bye to your husband and daughter, and have a girls' night out. Or spend a whole Saturday doing exactly what you want to do. Once a week, have a reading night. While your husband helps you get dinner or supervises homework duty, you curl up with one of those never-opened books for an hour or two.

It's great that you take "couple time" and "family time" vacations. They are great rejuvenators! For twenty-four hours, do what you want, when you want. Make sure you pamper yourself a bit— get a massage, a facial, or a pedicure to let someone take care of you! Don't feel guilty for a second. But if you do, just remember: When you take care of yourself, you take care of others better!

CHAPTER 8

The Energizing Power of Pleasure

When was the last time you experienced pure pleasure? (No, I'm not talking about sex here!) The kind you got as a kid as you played on the monkey bars or the ice-cream man handed you your favorite treat?

A swirl of happiness, enjoyment, and delight, pleasure is an essential part of a happy life. You know that old saying, "Stop to smell the roses"? Well, I live by it! I take time out of every day to simply appreciate the good things in my life, and life in general. Having morning coffee with my honey and reading the paper…preparing a delicious meal for my family and talking and laughing around the table…enjoying a girls' night out with my girlfriends—these are just a few of the simple pleasures that sweeten my life.

Pleasure revs up your energy. When you treat yourself to the small pleasures in life—a long walk, an evening of scrapbooking, a day at the beach—you are saying, *I love myself, and my happiness matters to me.* When it comes to emotional and mental fuel, happiness is the premium kind.

Of course, it's not always easy to pause amid the rush of life. (Boy, do I know it!) But the benefits are so worth that five or fifteen minutes. Taking time to savor the beauty around you does amazing things for your spirits and energy level.

The first step to pleasure is to live mindfully. When you're always on the go, there's no way to savor the scent of those roses. Your mind is always moving ahead to the next task on your to-do list.

One of the simplest ways to live in the now is to *breathe*. As silly as it sounds, slow, deep breaths help calm and focus your mind, and remind you of the simplest pleasure: life itself.

Living in the moment also means not being derailed by the small stuff. Sure, it's frustrating to sit in traffic for an hour. But do you want that petty annoyance to be your most vivid memory of the day? How much nicer to recall your child's hug and "I love you" that morning, or the pleasant twenty minutes you spent at the farmer's market, chatting with people and buying just-picked berries and tomatoes. For a few minutes, you put aside the details of life and enjoyed its delights.

You can add small pleasures to your life every day—they cost nothing, but enrich your life and spirit. This chapter is about how to open yourself to pleasure. Try the suggestions you find here and before long, you'll feel much happier and be a more energetic person.

Don't put off pleasure until tomorrow. Enjoy some today!

PEACE POCKET

Get into the Swing of Things!

Remember the joy you felt as a kid, flying high on that old tire swing or on the swing set? Relive it. The next time you take your kids or grandkids to the park, take the swing next to them. Feel the wind on your face and in your hair, stare up at the sky, and enjoy the pure pleasure of motion!

DECLUTTER YOUR LIFE

More than a century ago, the American philosopher Ralph Waldo Emerson praised the simple life. "Our life is frittered away by detail...Simplify, simplify." His words were never more true! To simplify your life is to make time to enjoy the important things. That's worth repeating: *You make the time.*

If you're like most people, you'd love more time to enjoy friends and family, and engage in activities that add meaning and satisfaction to your life. It's tough to maintain this serenity when you're working and caring for a family, too. You can't just declutter your home—you have to declutter your life! Once you let go of the things you don't really *need* to do, you'll be able to do the things that make life the beautiful, amazing adventure it was meant to be. Here are four ways to start the decluttering process.

1. **Stop trying to keep up with the Joneses.** Do you really need a bigger house, a new bedroom set, a plasma TV? Do your kids really need the newest high-tech gadget? There's nothing wrong with wanting the finer things in life, or wanting to give your kids the best that money can buy. As the old saying goes, though, money can't buy happiness. When you truly notice, and appreciate, the simple pleasures of life, and pass them on to your children, you may find that they're more satisfying than material possessions.

2. **Give yourself time to breathe.** It's wonderful to volunteer your time to community and church projects. If you give too much, however, you'll spend all your time rushing from one commitment to the next. In doing for others, are you cheating yourself of the pleasures of life? If you're overcommitted, rethink your priorities. Keep only the most important commitments and bow out of those that fall

lower on your priority list. Spend your newfound free time on activities that will bring you true happiness.

3. **Live according to your values.** Values are those things that matter deeply to you. Some examples include worship, creativity, dependability, tolerance, and trustworthiness. Only you know what your values are, and whether you're living by them. Give some thought to the beliefs that you hold dear. If you're living in conflict with them, you may feel so tense or blue that there's no room for pleasure. Follow your heart, and life will become fun and full again.

4. **Tame your inner control freak.** Trying to control life isn't pleasurable. In fact, it's downright frustrating! Think of how much nicer life could be if you stopped trying to control what others do, say, or think, or the outcome of some aspect of your home or work life. For one thing, you'd probably enjoy the journey that is life much more. When you stop trying to control things, you open yourself to pleasure, along with new opportunities.

PEACE POCKET

Do an Old-Time Sunday Dinner

If you love to cook but have the local pizza place on speed-dial, clear a space in your schedule and cook an old-fashioned Sunday meal. It doesn't have to be fancy. If you know how to bake bread, how about a fresh-baked loaf with a hearty, slow-simmered soup? Or roast chicken with fresh veggies and homemade mashed potatoes? There is little more pleasurable than preparing a meal, then sitting down to enjoy it with the people you love.

100 SIMPLE PLEASURES

Pleasure is like cinnamon: a little goes a long way, and it only takes a dash to spice things up!

Simple pleasures are life's treasures. One of my greatest pleasures is to sip my morning coffee slowly, enjoying its steam and bold aroma, as I read the paper with my husband. When I finish the horoscope, I'm energized and ready to tackle my day. I sprinkle little pleasures throughout the rest of my day to keep me going, or just stop to enjoy those simple joys that come my way. By bedtime, I've had a pretty pleasurable day.

What simple pleasures could you add to *your* day? The list below gives you a starting point, but I encourage you to find your own. Make them happen, or—when they happen to you—recognize them as gifts in an otherwise ordinary day and take a moment to savor them. (I'm hoping that just reading this list will give you a lift!) The more simple pleasures you can add to each day, the more you'll enjoy *every* day.

1. Sleeping late on a rainy weekend morning.
2. Telling a long, complicated, but great joke—perfectly.
3. Finding a favorite shirt you'd forgotten about in the back of your closet.
4. Reminiscing about old times.
5. Sharing a good laugh.
6. Holding hands with a child.
7. Making someone smile.
8. Scuffling through a pile of autumn leaves.
9. Laughing so hard your tummy muscles hurt.
10. A hot shower after a long day.
11. Tiny, cute living things: puppies, babies, kittens.
12. Going to an afternoon movie, alone.
13. Blowing bubbles with a child.

14. Exchanging smiles with an attractive stranger.
15. The feeling you get when someone forgives you, or you forgive someone.
16. Falling asleep in the sun.
17. Waking up and realizing you don't have to get up for hours.
18. Swinging on a swing (especially an old-fashioned tire swing!).
19. Making bread or cookies.
20. Getting lost in a great book.
21. Sipping hot chocolate during a snowstorm.
22. Using a towel fresh from the dryer.
23. Sitting around the table, telling family stories.
24. Coffee in bed with the Sunday paper.
25. Watching a child romp with his dog.
26. A picnic in the park.
27. Taking a long, rambling walk.
28. Eating fresh-baked bread with lots of butter.
29. Sitting on your front porch watching lightning in the distance.
30. Leafing through your high school yearbook.
31. Renting a tearjerker and indulging your emotions, with a bowl of popcorn.
32. Looking at old family pictures.
33. Splashing through a mud puddle.
34. Making gingerbread men for Christmas.
35. Eating all the marshmallows out of a box of Lucky Charms.
36. Sitting on the couch watching your lit-up Christmas tree in the dark.
37. Giving the dog a bath.
38. Dipping sun-warmed strawberries in sugar.
39. Attending a potluck dinner and bringing your own covered dish.

40. Sitting in a deck chair in early summer, watching the sun set.
41. Getting a kite airborne and letting a child hold the string.
42. Putting the last piece of a thousand-piece jigsaw puzzle into place.
43. Picking your own apples, strawberries, or pumpkins.
44. Going bowling on a Saturday night.
45. Watching your kids sleep (finally!) after a long day.
46. Checking tasks off your to-do list, one by one.
47. Watching fireflies wink on a summer evening.
48. Trick-or-treating with your kids or grandkids.
49. Eating just-picked veggies from your own garden.
50. Sleeping naked with a cool breeze blowing over you.
51. Watching your partner sleep.
52. Watching cartoons with your kids on Saturday morning.
53. Waking up to a tidy kitchen.
54. Wandering around the local farmer's market.
55. Dedicating a love song on the radio, knowing your loved one is listening.
56. Taking a long, decadent nap on Saturday afternoon.
57. Playing cards or a board game with family or friends.
58. Swinging in a hammock on a beautiful day.
59. Sitting on the sand at the edge of the shore, letting the ocean lap on your toes.
60. Breezing through the supermarket checkout line after work.
61. Getting a call from an old friend, out of the blue.
62. Finding $10 in the washer or dryer.
63. Finding a parking space right in front.
64. Packing for a vacation.
65. Getting your hair washed before a haircut.
66. Spying the first daffodils of spring.
67. Being safe and warm at home during a blizzard.

68. That peaceful feeling after a long, good cry.
69. Going to a big wedding and dancing all night.
70. Being the first one up on a Sunday morning.
71. Crying because something wonderful happened.
72. The comfortable silence between you and an old friend.
73. Slipping into clean, soft pajamas.
74. Hearing the soothing rush of a spring or waterfall.
75. Having someone brush your hair.
76. The sight of a long, green field of corn.
77. The smell of rain in summer.
78. Making a sand castle with your child or grandchild.
79. Finding a parking meter with an hour still on it.
80. Driving in the rain at night with someone you love.
81. Setting down your suitcases and being happy to be home after a trip.
82. Holding hands with your partner.
83. The first lick of an ice-cream cone.
84. Helping to give a baby a bath, or watching her at bath time.
85. Waking up to your cat or dog nestled against you.
86. Seeing the clouds below you when riding in an airplane.
87. Making someone else's day brighter by paying a sincere compliment.
88. Turning on the radio to find the station playing your favorite song.
89. Sunlight on a clean kitchen floor.
90. Sitting around a campfire, talking and making s'mores.
91. Hosting, or attending, a summer barbecue.
92. The smell of autumn—wood smoke and leaves.
93. Watching your child sing in a school pageant or perform in a school play.
    Waking up early and hearing the birds chirping.
    'tepping into the shower after a hard workout.

96. Blowing out *all* your birthday candles.
97. Watching the groom kiss the bride.
98. Finding a pot holder or pencil holder you made as a kid.
99. Snuggling into fresh, line-dried bedsheets.
100. Being told you have beautiful eyes.

YOUR DAILY PLEASURE PLAN

Childhood is a time of pleasure—and energy. Everything is new, fresh, and children revel in it all. They have little sense of time, and live in each moment happily and fully. And we adults should live the same way! These four steps can help you add more pleasure—and energy—to each and every day.

1. **Ask yourself what gives you pleasure.** Have you ever really considered this question? Now's the time! Quick: Write down three things that you do simply because they're fun or make you feel good.

    1. _____

    2. _____

    3. _____

    No, you're not "too busy" to add pleasure to your life. As the list above shows, many pleasures can be measured in minutes, or even seconds!

    What's on your list? Your daily walk? Playing with your dog in the backyard? Sharing a meal with extended family, or a cup of tea with a friend? Hiking in the woods or ambling by the water?

Plan your own moment of pleasure today—literally put it on your to-do list. Take it seriously—make sure you check it off every day. Pay attention to the pleasure you feel. Live in that moment, and relive it later. In fact, if you build up a "pleasure bank" of memories to draw on when you're feeling blue, they can often get you through!

2. **Imagine yourself as a five-year-old.** Pleasure begins with loving and valuing yourself—and that means taking care of yourself. So for at least fifteen minutes a day, give yourself the same loving attention and care you would give a small child.

   Feed yourself good, healthy meals and snacks every few hours. Set up regular times for play (exercise) and bedtime, and don't let anything disrupt those, either. Make regular "playdates" with friends. Take yourself to the doctor and the dentist. When you care for yourself the same way you would your own child, your niece or nephew, or your best friend's child, you're bound to have as much energy as they do.

3. **To find pleasure, depend on your senses.** Very often, they work as your pleasure detectors! For example, on your walk, focus on the warmth of the day, the chirping of birds, the crunch and smell of the fall leaves under your feet. (Try to avoid using unhealthy food as a pleasure, though. While eating a doughnut might give you momentary enjoyment, you sure won't feel that way ten seconds after the last bite!) Look for pleasure, and you will find it—and energy along with it.

4. **Learn to be spontaneous.** I know it's not easy—I've got a schedule and obligations, too. But it's so important to learn to enjoy life on the fly, in the moment. Pleasure doesn't have to last long to be energizing. In fact, you can experience it in seconds, if you go with the flow.

ENERGY MAKEOVER!

RITA VALENTI, 60
HOMETOWN: FLUSHING, NEW YORK
OCCUPATION: ACCOUNTING

Rita Valenti told me she knows exactly what drains her energy: a sedentary lifestyle. "I get up each morning at 4:30 AM, do a few chores, and am on the road by 6 AM so I arrive at work by 7," she wrote me. Although New York City has a great mass-transit system, she explains, driving reduces her three-hour round-trip commute to about twenty minutes each way, so it just makes sense to drive.

Once at work, Rita says, she sits for eight to ten hours a day. "I get up only to go to the copy machine, the ladies' room, or the conference room. My job is stressful—I face constant deadlines and there are millions of dollars at stake. You'd need a person and a half to handle my workload. Unfortunately, there's only one: me! On the positive side, I work with a friendly little group, with whom I usually have lunch."

Rita typically leaves the office late. "I always hope to get to the gym, but that hope dwindles as I realize how exhausted I am," she says. Once at home, her only "exercise" is to move around her small kitchen to make dinner. Then she sits to eat it, usually at the television.

She follows a fairly healthy diet, because she has high cholesterol and high blood pressure. "Still, I could lose about thirty pounds," she writes. "I have a gym membership, and I haven't gone in ages, but I won't give it up—I guess I hold out hope that I'll find the time or inspiration to work out again."

After dinner, Rita takes a seat behind her computer—"that is, if I don't nod out in my recliner at 7:30." She adds that her sleep habits are poor—she goes to bed between 11 PM and midnight, but if she falls asleep after dinner, she wakes at 10:30 and is up for hours.

Rita tells me that she considers herself a fairly happy, positive person (good!). "Although I don't have many close friends to socialize with, I do have many interests, like writing and photography," she says. "I am also close to my siblings, although we're scattered all over the country." She has a house in the mountains and loves to garden there, as well as cook and can, but admits that she rarely gets away, as her sister's eighteen-year-old daughter lives with her (she became a part of Rita's household four years ago). "I also used to meditate, but it's difficult to find the time for that," Rita says. "I know there's more to life than my stale routine. I just need the energy to find it!"

Rita, when I read your e-mail, I thought: *It's funny how sitting, an activity at which you never break a sweat, can leave you so exhausted!* Fortunately, there's much you can do to add movement to your desk job—and your life.

First, start your day with my morning stretch—it takes just five minutes, and you have five minutes to feel better, right? Since you already have an interest in meditation, this routine is the perfect opportunity to energize for the day ahead. At work, do my afternoon stretch to get that blood pumping and stretch cramped, oxygen-deprived muscles.

Because you're a city girl, you have to make the time, or create an opportunity, to move! If there's a neighborhood park nearby, walk at lunchtime. Ask your co-workers if they'd like to join you. You'd have fun, get regular exercise, and shake off work-related stress to boot. If there's no nearby park, walk at a brisk pace for a couple of blocks.

As strange as this sounds, try not to sit for more than ten minutes at a time after you eat dinner. I know you're tired, but as you say, it's a full day of sitting that tires you out! Make it a challenge. Pace while you talk on the phone. Whether you're watching TV or surfing the Internet, get up and do leg lifts at every commercial (or every ten minutes if you're on the computer). You'll feel so much better! If you really need to nap, set your alarm or oven timer for fifteen minutes and catnap. You'll sleep so much deeper!

Speaking of sleep: Up at 4 AM, bed at 11 PM...you do realize that you're awake nineteen hours a day, don't you? No wonder you're exhausted! Sleep is not merely a time-out from your busy life; it is essential for good health, especially cardiovascular health.

If you truly want more energy, you'll need to make changes. Sleep an hour later in the morning, or go to bed earlier. Yes, you'll need to let some things fall by the wayside. But at the end of the day, what means more: that you accomplished one extra errand, or that you did something good for yourself?

You say you're in a rut. Well, ruts don't spark energy. Novelty does. Shake things up! While you can't change much about your weekday routine, your weekends are all yours.

For starters, invite your niece to your house in the mountains once in a while. Offer to teach her to garden, cook, or can. It's a way to bond, and to pass on traditional skills to a new generation. Even if she declines your invitation, drive up yourself. (She's an adult, after all!) Surround yourself with nature. Engage in activities that are meaningful to you. Since you enjoy photography, why not take your camera along on a walk outside? You'll rejuvenate your spirit, which will, in turn, reignite your energy. When you can't get away, get involved in activities that engage your mind and body—a writing group, a photography club, or a local walking group. And since you already belong to a gym, why not work out on the weekends, when you're home? If you go at least twice a week, then it's worth the price of membership. And those workouts will definitely impact your energy levels!

There you have it. Now go forth and shake up that "stale routine" you mentioned. Once you begin to honor your needs (and sleep! Don't forget to sleep!), you'll start to see a difference in your energy level. Just think about what you'd love to do with your free time—if you had any—then do it!

CHAPTER 9

Power Up at Midlife!

As I write this book, I just turned fifty-three, and honestly I feel like I'm thirty-five. Thank God I have the energy to do everything I love to do, and that's what I hope for you, too!

But of course, at this age, I have noticed a few changes in my body. I have hot flashes and night sweats now and again. Sometimes, when I wake up in the middle of the night to pee, I find that it takes me a while to fall back asleep. I have chosen not to use hormone replacement therapy. I am dealing with these midlife changes naturally…by doing more stretching and strength training, watching my diet more carefully, and taking a few supplements to ease my symptoms and protect my health. I'm doing the best I can, naturally, and so far, it seems to be working!

The thing about perimenopause, though, is that each woman experiences it differently. While some women, like me, pass through it with few symptoms, one of the most common symptoms is fatigue. You may feel generally "worn out"—you struggle against daytime drowsiness, and may even sneak in an afternoon nap. You may also notice more "down" days, feel snappish, or have a harder time managing your normal routine.

Here are some reasons why you may be exhausted in perimenopause: Changes in estrogen levels can make it tough to sleep and/or sleep soundly, and may contribute to those negative moods. Some women in perimenopause are diagnosed with low thyroid, fibromyalgia, or chronic fatigue syndrome, all of which can leave you wiped out. A less-than-healthy diet, a couch-potato lifestyle, and chronic stress can contribute to midlife fatigue as well.

If you're over forty and always tired, perimenopause may be a factor. But you don't have to take this fatigue lying down (although you might love to!). There's plenty you can do to rev up that energy and recharge those batteries, and I'm here to cheer you on!

To regain your energy, you must first take back your power. Laughter really can help, which is why you see so many T-shirts, coffee mugs, and other fun gift items that make light of perimenopause. (I recently saw a coffee mug that said, IT'S NOT YOU. NO, WAIT. IT IS.)

The second step is to understand what about perimenopause can potentially sap your energy, so you can plug that leak! So in this chapter, we're first going to look at some of the symptoms you may be experiencing. Then I'll give you some suggestions for what you can do to alleviate those symptoms so that you can fight fatigue, get a decent night's sleep, and feel better all around.

THE CHANGE BEFORE THE CHANGE

What we call menopause is actually made up of several different stages; the earliest is perimenopause. This is when those new symptoms begin: irregular periods, spotting, night sweats and/or hot flashes. Technically, menopause occurs the moment our ovaries run out of eggs. Did you know that every woman starts out with a lifetime supply of eggs? Menstruation, in which the body sheds the uterine lining to prepare for the fertilization of an egg, is no longer necessary when there are no more eggs.

Menopause is when menstruation stops for good. No one can predict exactly when it will happen—although some women can become menopausal as early as age thirty-five, on average women reach menopause at fifty-one.

The period between perimenopause and the permanent end of menstrual periods can last for years. During that time, you could experience an emotional roller coaster—you feel alternately moody, sad, and out of control. These unpredictable emotions occur because when you run out of eggs, you also stop producing the sex hormones estrogen, progesterone, and testosterone. Many women also suffer less-than-comfortable physical side effects, such as hot flashes, fatigue, vaginal dryness, and insomnia. If this is happening to you, you are definitely not alone!

The good news? You can reduce the symptoms of menopause with exercise and healthy eating. That's right! Regular workouts can lessen the severity and frequency of hot flashes and night sweats, and can fight depression and fatigue. Also, to stay in shape as you age, it's vital to maintain a healthy lifestyle during menopause. Now is as important a time as ever to eat right, get fit, and do all you can to feel great—and I'm here to help you do it!

HOW YOUR PHYSICAL ENERGY MAY CHANGE

Perimenopause can take up a *lot* of extra energy. That's no surprise—after all, you're dealing with significant hormonal changes that affect not just your energy level, but virtually every other aspect of your physical and emotional well-being! Not to mention the fact that, as a woman, you don't get a free pass just because your hormones are all over the place. You likely still have a lot on your plate—work, kids, household chores, and everything else you did *before* your hormones went crazy on top of it! Here's what you may be experiencing now.

Fatigue

You have a household to run, a family or an aging parent to care for, and (maybe) a job outside your home that takes a big chunk of your time. Your hectic life alone is enough to drain your energy. Add the fatigue of perimenopause, however, and you may experience the "crashing fatigue" that hits many women in this period of their lives. Crashing fatigue is a commonly used phrase that describes the extreme fatigue many women in perimenopause deal with.

Sometimes this type of fatigue is caused by insomnia (more about this in a second). However, your perimenopausal body also makes less of the male sex hormone testosterone. (Yes, women's bodies make this, too!) Although we make a minuscule amount of testosterone, it's this hormone that keeps women energized. There is good news: Many women regain their energy once their periods stop for good.

Trouble Sleeping

Boy, do I know this one! Occasionally, I wake up with night sweats and have to change my jammies, and then have trouble getting back to sleep. Other friends have told me that they wake up in the wee hours of the morning and are unable to fall back asleep, or start awake with their hearts pounding. The day after "those nights," I'm a big believer in taking a fifteen- or twenty-minute catnap!

There's no doubt that insomnia and/or disrupted sleep affects your daytime energy level, as you may already know. Blame hormonal fluctuations for that daytime drowsiness. In perimenopause, your body circulates less estrogen, which triggers symptoms— including night sweats, headaches, and nausea—that can make it harder to fall and stay asleep.

Stress also contributes to poor sleep in perimenopause, as do hormone-induced fluctuations in your body temperature. Even if you don't *feel* a hot flash, your body temperature may have risen to the point where it wakes you up. It will take time for your temperature to fall again, which makes it difficult to fall back to sleep. Thankfully, you don't have to forgo sleep—there are a number of things that may help you fall and stay asleep, which we'll get to later in this chapter.

Weight Gain

Is it getting harder for you to maintain a healthy weight or to lose weight? Me too. These days, whenever I enjoy eating a little too much, I notice that my middle gets a little poochy. (Ten years ago, any overindulgence showed up on my thighs!)

Yes, hormones certainly play a role in midlife weight gain, but they're not the whole story. You may not eat as well, and turn to comfort foods to ease perimenopausal symptoms. Or perhaps your daily workouts have dwindled, which means you lose calorie-burning muscle.

Speaking of muscle: If your weight is creeping up, hit those weights! It's an unfortunate fact that aging promotes the replacement of muscle with fat, which means we burn fewer calories. Muscle works miracles on your metabolism. Why? Because muscle burns more calories than fat does…up to a hundred more calories a day! My twenty-minute workout in chapter 12 will firm and tone those muscles, and do great things for your weight, energy, and spirits to boot.

POSSIBLE CHANGES IN YOUR MENTAL AND EMOTIONAL ENERGY

Did you ever see those T-shirts made especially for women in perimenopause? Many poke gentle fun at the emotional and mental changes that can accompany this phase of a woman's life. (My personal favorite: MENOPAUSE IS MY EXCUSE AND I'M STICKING TO IT!) Here's what you may be feeling now.

Brain Fog

"Where did I put my keys?" "Where did I leave my glasses?" "It's on the tip of my tongue..."

Sound familiar? Unfortunately, forgetfulness or "brain fog" is common in perimenopause. You may feel mentally "fuzzy," cross the room to get or do something and forget why, or find it difficult to focus or concentrate. While lost in brain fog, it's not likely that you'll be a bundle of energy. In fact, some women describe brain fog as a "drugged" feeling.

While these symptoms are annoying, they're usually not serious: For most perimenopausal women, these are temporary conditions caused by (you guessed it) hormonal changes and stress.

Insomnia, or sleep challenges, is a big culprit in this mental fuzziness—it's hard to think when you haven't slept well in days. It's also true that decreasing estrogen levels at this time of life affect our brain function and memory.

You'll take heart, though, from the conclusions of this study. Starting in 1996, researchers from Rush–Presbyterian–St. Luke's Medical Center in Chicago gave memory tests over the course of years to perimenopausal women. Their conclusion: Women with brain fog don't need to worry. The confusion and memory loss many women feel in perimenopause will eventually clear...just like fog!

Moodiness

An estimated 10 to 20 percent of women in perimenopause experience mood changes. Some feel sad, anxious, or angry, experience mood swings, or get irritable or tearful. Needless to say, this kind of emotional roller coaster probably won't do much for a woman's energy level.

If you've noticed these kinds of symptoms, don't blame yourself! It's thought that some women may be more vulnerable to hormone-related mood changes than others. Be kind to yourself, and remember that this, too, shall pass.

To fight back against moodiness, lace up your sneakers and get that daily thirty minutes of exercise. One of the biggest reasons I work out is that exercise acts as my mental filter: It filters out any grouchiness or tension I might feel. I'd bet that exercise will act as your filter, too!

GET BACK YOUR GET-UP-AND-GO!

Now that you know a bit about why you're feeling tired, let's look at what you can do about it. Yes, there are lots of ways you can ramp up your energy and feel years younger. While not all of these lifestyle changes may work for you, I'd bet that many will—and before long, your energy will come roaring back!

Revitalize with Diet

- **Get those Daily Dozen into your diet!** At midlife, it's more important than ever to pass up processed foods for fresh, whole foods. Keep it simple: Every day, eat three fruits, three veggies, three servings of protein, two servings of a healthy grain like brown rice or oatmeal, and one serving of a healthy fat, such as olive oil, nuts, or avocado. I call this the Daily Dozen, and if you team it with thirty minutes of exercise, you'll find it much easier to maintain a healthy weight (or lose weight) and fight any unpleasant effects of perimenopause. The cleaner you eat, the better it is for your body, your mood, and your attitude!

- **Fill up on fiber.** I'm always touting the benefits of a fiber-rich diet, but it's especially important for women at midlife. Besides keeping you "regular," a diet rich in fiber can significantly lower your risk of heart disease and can drive down high blood cholesterol levels. It can even act as a natural appetite suppressant, filling you up faster and for longer, which will help you keep those portion sizes under control. Crunchy apples, hearty beans, and creamy oatmeal fit the bill.

- **Keep a food diary.** Research has repeatedly shown that people who track what they eat lose more weight than those who don't track. But there's another benefit—tracking what you eat along with your symptoms will help you identify food triggers. You'll learn whether specific foods or types of food (spicy foods, caffeinated beverages, what have you) cause you discomfort so you can avoid them.

Re-Energize with Exercise

- **Stay active!** The first five minutes of a workout can be the toughest, even for me…but oh, the feeling after you're done! When you exercise, your brain releases endorphins—feel-good chemicals that improve your mood. So if you feel sad or anxious, lace up those sneakers and walk it off. Other bonuses: That thirty minutes of physical activity also burns calories and may control hot flashes—and it will definitely help you sleep better at night.

- **Exercise earlier in the day.** Many women, especially if they work outside the home, can only squeeze in a workout in the evening. If you're one of them, and it works for you, keep doing it! Just make sure you're done at least three hours before bed. Sleep experts have found that exercise too close to bedtime can rev you up, which can leave you tossing and turning. If possible, I strongly suggest working out in the morning. Personally, a morning workout works for me—when I'm home, I'm up and exercising with my honey even before the kids are up. That early-morning workout boosts my energy and mood all day, and best of all, I don't have to worry all day about when I'll have time to squeeze in those thirty minutes.

Recharge with Lifestyle Changes

- **Try to reduce stress.** Not only because stress can trigger hot flashes and other uncomfortable symptoms of menopause, but because stress is hard on your heart and your body in general—and now more than ever, you really need to take care of your health! Meditation, deep breathing, and progressive relaxation techniques can be very helpful, especially if stress or anxiety tend to keep you up. And if your stress is caused by an issue in a relationship, try talking out what's bothering you with that person.

- **Eliminate triggers.** Caffeine and alcohol can interfere with sleep—I can tell you that from personal experience! I love my red wine, but if I have more than one glass these days, I know I won't sleep well that night. (I have to have a *really* good reason to have two!) Forgo that glass of wine with dinner if you have hot flashes, too. Alcohol can triggers those blasts of heat, as can caffeine, nicotine, and hot drinks.

- **Adjust the temperature.** Hot flashes and night sweats can really mess up your sleep. To combat the sensation of heat, keep your nighttime environment cooler than usual. Yes, you can turn down the heat, but you can also use a fan and trade in flannel jammies for cotton. (I took the down comforter out of my beautiful duvet cover, and now use the duvet as a pretty bedspread—problem solved!)

TOO TIRED FOR SEX? WHAT TO DO

Decreased sex drive is not uncommon among women in their forties and fifties. It is often related to stress, hormone fluctuations, depression, and a variety of other causes. In perimenopausal women specifically, it may be caused by painful sex. After all, who wants to do it if it hurts!

Each person's sex drive is different, so it's hard to find a definition for a "low" sex drive. The best way to think about it is that the desire to have sex is not as strong as it used to be. Women who are in touch with their sexuality will readily recognize this change in themselves.

When one partner has a higher or lower sex drive than the other, it can create sexual challenges for both of them. If this should happen, communication is important. Talk openly with your partner about your sexual needs and feelings; discussing sexual fantasies may also boost your desire for sex. Try to enjoy intimate activities together that do not involve sex, like cuddling or massage. Speak to your health-care provider as well (don't be shy!). He or she may be able to adjust medications or try hormone therapy.

ASK FOR A HELPING HAND!

If you're like most women, you're the primary caretaker—the "go-to" girl. That's not likely to change, but what can change is your reluctance to ask for help. To re-energize, ask for some assistance—or take the bull by the horns and give yourself a hand!

- **At work.** Do late hours or on-the-job stress drain your energy? At least a few nights a week, make it a point to leave the office on time—and don't take work home. And take the occasional "mental health day" if you need it, too.

- **At home.** Can't fall or stay asleep? Overwhelmed by your to-do list? Ask your partner or kids to make dinner a few nights during the week so you can catch a twenty-minute nap. You work hard—you deserve it! (Just don't nap too long, or you'll have a hard time falling asleep at bedtime.)

IF YOU'RE STILL TIRED...

If you have tried some or all of these recommendations without success, don't give up! Schedule a doctor's visit to discuss your options. This is a good idea if your blue mood lingers more than a week or two, or if you toss and turn night after night. She or he may suggest that you be evaluated for other problems, such as low thyroid function or obstructive sleep apnea, a major cause of daytime sleepiness. (If you snore, you should definitely tell your doctor!) Depending on your individual situation, your doctor also can talk to you about other treatments that can help you reclaim your vitality in perimenopause.

Here are a few options to discuss with your doctor:

- **Herbal remedies.** With your doctor's okay, you might try black cohosh, an herb that has been shown to reduce menopausal symptoms for some women. Also, valerian, a mild, non-addictive herb, has a long history as a sleep aid.
- **A snoring machine.** Continuous positive airway pressure (CPAP) is a treatment that can ease breathing at night in menopausal women with fatigue and obstructive sleep apnea, a condition of disordered nighttime breathing.
- **Prescription medications.** Your doctor can help you decide whether medications could help with symptoms such as hot flashes, insomnia, or mood issues.

One more thing: Midlife can be an amazing time. At this stage of my life, my priorities are firmly in place, and I'm freer than ever to honor them. I spend time with the people I want to spend time with, and do the projects I want with the people I like to work with. You may find that, with your kids older or even out of the nest, you have the freedom to go back to school, learn a new hobby, or offer your time to a cause you believe in…you call the shots!

So spread your wings! This stage of life is a gift—a chance to rediscover yourself and your passions. You'll need energy for that— and if you take care of your body, engage your mind, and nourish your spirit, you can recapture that youthful vitality. Remember— forty is the new thirty, and fifty is the new forty. So go for it!

ENERGY MAKEOVER!

ANGELA BAITY, 50
HOMETOWN: INMAN, SOUTH CAROLINA
OCCUPATION: WOMEN'S COUNSELOR

When I read Angela Baity's e-mail, I knew I had to reach out to her. She has been having a tough time with "The Change."

"Everyone always says that 'fifty is the new forty,' but it hasn't turned out quite that way for me," Angela writes. "All my life, I was a strong, sexy, vibrant woman who enjoyed life. When I reached this milestone, however, things changed. My body didn't seem like mine anymore, and depression took hold."

As a result of this hormonal roller coaster, Angela has gained ten pounds and suffers with hot flashes and night sweats. The severity of the hot flashes seems to depend on the amount of emotional stress she's experienced that day, she notes. "And between my mood and financial worries, I have my share!" Because of the night sweats, she gets about three hours of sleep a night.

Her libido has changed, too. "I have almost no desire, which is not like me," she says. "Although my husband tries to be understanding, it has caused problems. I've heard that natural hormone replacement helps with the hot flashes, night sweats, and libido, but I went for a consultation and the cost was prohibitive."

Angela does eat a healthy diet of whole foods and watches her portions. However, those ten pounds won't budge. "It's not low thyroid—I've been tested for that, and the tests came back normal."

Angela thinks that her weight gain is due to the fact that she can't exercise without pain. "I used to love to walk and ride my bike, but joint pain and exhaustion prevent it now," she writes. "I *want* to exercise, but my motivation and energy last only for a day, and then the exhaustion creeps in again. If I manage to get a walk or a bike ride in, my entire body is sore and my joints hurt the next day."

A friend of Angela's, who happens to be a massage therapist, gives her the occasional massage (that must feel heavenly!). Her friend mentioned that Angela might want to be tested for fibro-myalgia, and she's scheduled a doctor's appointment to find out.

In the meantime, though, her energy and zest for life have taken a hit. "Just a few years ago, I felt so vibrant and enjoyed life—I loved to swim and work in my flower garden, but I can't enjoy those activities now," says Angela. "I have a close friend who lives about forty-five minutes away. We see each other every few weeks, and talk on the phone often. She's been a lifesaver.

"I pray every day that my energy returns. I want to find my way back to the woman I used to be, so I can help other women, but I need some help myself. Please help—I want to live again!"

*   *   *

Angela, I *promise*: That strong, sexy, vibrant woman is alive and well within you. Though it may take some time to find her again, I'm here to help you do it!

Let's leave the ten pounds alone for now. As frustrating as they may be, your other symptoms should be addressed first—by a doctor. And good for you for calling your doctor, because the pain and exhaustion you describe fit the description of fibromyalgia, characterized by exhaustion, tender joints, reduced exercise tolerance, and depression. Although only a doctor can diagnose you, if you do have fibromyalgia, the sooner you begin treatment, the sooner you and your doctor, together, can begin to manage your symptoms.

The hormonal fluctuations of midlife have also been associated with lack of energy—some women call it crashing fatigue. Besides, if you average three hours of sleep a night, and have hot flashes and night sweats on top of it, your energy is bound to take a hit! You may want to ask your doctor about natural progesterone cream and "women's herbs" such as black cohosh. Also, since I turned fifty, I take twelve hundred milligrams of fish oil, in capsule form, every day. Not only do those omega-3 fatty acids help protect your heart and overall health, research suggests that they may help ease depression, too! I also recommend adding ground flaxseed to your diet. I grind my own and put a tablespoon in my cereal or spaghetti sauce every day. Available at most natural food stores, all of these remedies can offer relief at an affordable price. Talk to your doctor before you take them, though, so they don't interact with any prescription or over-the-counter medications you currently take.

Another way to revive your flagging energy: Drink lots of water. Hydration definitely keeps your energy high, and I swear by it! Talk to your doctor about strength training, too—it's especially wonderful for women in midlife. Check out my twenty-minute workout in chapter 12. If your doctor approves, but you find you can't do the whole twenty minutes, do the first part, at minimum. Even those ten minutes will brighten your mood and tone your body all over!

We all follow our own paths on the journey of life, and sometimes the passage gets rocky. One thing that always helps me, as simple as it sounds, is to count my blessings. You have a loving, supportive husband, close friends, and a career that you love. That's a lot! As hard as it may be, turn those negative feelings into positive action, such as asking for help. Follow your doctor's advice, and above all be kind to yourself! Treat yourself to little indulgences (a warm bath, a bouquet of fresh flowers) and lean on the people who love you. We all grow older, but when we stay positive, our spirits can remain forever young!

PART THREE
HIGH-ENERGY LIVING

CHAPTER 10

Your Personal Energy Plan Worksheet

This worksheet has an important purpose: to get you to consider your habits, and schedule, with a fresh pair of eyes. Sometimes we get so overwhelmed and wrapped up in the big picture, we don't look at the details. Well, the details are important here. This worksheet will help you do a thorough analysis of your lifestyle, showing you exactly where you could make positive, energizing changes that fit *your* schedule, habits, and lifestyle.

Before you begin the worksheet, answer this question: *Is my fatigue so bad, or my mood so blue, that I wonder if there's a physical or emotional cause?* If you answered yes, put down your pen, pick up the phone, and schedule an appointment with your doctor. Yes, right now! She or he may want to test for conditions that can cause fatigue, such as hypothyroidism, fibromyalgia, anemia, or clinical depression.

Devote as much time as you can to this worksheet—at least thirty minutes. The more thoughtful and detailed your answers, the more personalized your plan will be. If you don't have enough space to write (or if you just don't like writing in books), feel free to use a separate piece of paper. Make the time—we're talking about changing your life here! The time and energy you'll save going forward are worth it, and so are you.

PART I: *YOUR LIFE RIGHT NOW*

1. During the week, what time do you go to bed, and when do you wake up?

    _____

2. On weekends, what time do you go to bed, and when do you wake up?

    _____

3. What part of the day do you typically have the least energy—morning, midafternoon, after work?

    _____

4. List the times during the week, including the weekend, that you typically watch TV (for example, "One hour of TV, Monday through Friday, from 9 to 10 PM and Saturdays 8 to 9 AM").

    _____

    _____

    _____

    _____

5. List the times during the week, including the weekend, that you typically spend on the computer (for example, "Two

hours of Internet time, Monday through Friday, from 8 to 10 PM").

_____

_____

_____

_____

6. What are your standing weekday obligations (church, volunteer organizations, meetings, carpooling, kids' activities, et cetera)? Number them in order of priority, from most to least pressing.

_____

_____

_____

_____

7. What are your standing weekend obligations (yard work, taking children to sports or lessons, et cetera)? Number them in order of priority, from most to least pressing.

_____

_____

_____

_____

8. If you work outside the home: How long is your daily commute to work?

_____

9. What time of day would you be most likely to get thirty minutes of uninterrupted time to yourself?

_____

PART 2: *DARE TO DELEGATE!*

Considering the weekday and weekend obligations in the previous section, list those that you could delegate right now. Be honest—include anything that you *could* ask your partner, your teen or adult child, a parent, or a friend to do, even though you know you can do them better or "the way they should be done." After each task or project, list the approximate amount of time you've freed up in your day, week, or month.

1. _____

2. _____

3. _____

4. _____

5. _____

PART 3: *YOUR GO-TO EMERGENCY ENERGY BOOSTERS AND DE-STRESSORS*

1. Page through this book and list the three "Revive in 5!" tips you're most likely to use.

   a. _____

   b. _____

   c. _____

2. Now list three "Peace Pockets" that appeal to you. If you've been inspired to come up with your own, feel free to list those as well or instead.

    a. _____

    b. _____

    c. _____

3. If you've come up with any energy boosters or de-stressors on your own, list them here.

    _____
    _____

4. List one "get me through" saying that you would be likely to repeat to yourself when you're under stress (Serenity Prayer, "this too shall pass," and the like).

    _____
    _____

5. List two people you could call when you're at the end of your rope.

    _____
    _____

6. List two to three things you could do with half an hour of personal time per day.

    _____
    _____
    _____

7. List two to three things you could do with an hour of
    personal time per week.

    _____

    _____

    _____

8. List two to three things you could do with a whole day, or
    weekend, of personal time.

    _____

    _____

    _____

PART 4: *CALCULATE THE TIME YOU'VE SAVED!*

Using the information in parts 1 and 2, add up the time you could
shave from your schedule. Look carefully at the tasks or projects
you could delegate, the last items on your weekday and weekend
obligations, and the time you spend watching TV and using the
Internet.

1. Time I would save delegating projects or tasks during the
    week or on weekends:

    _____

2. Time I would save if I gave up the last priority on my
    weekday and/or weekend obligation list:

    _____

3. Time I would save if I halved my TV and Internet time per
    week:

    _____

With that time, pick personal time activities from your lists in part 3.

- My picks:

_____

_____

_____

PART 5: *START SAVING ENERGY!*

Armed with the information in parts 1–4, you're ready to create your personal energy makeover. Follow the simple instructions below. If you have a job outside the home, or if you care for your children at home, add "work" or "mothering" to indicate a large block of time. To cope with stress or fatigue, use the "Revive in 5!" or "Peace Pockets" you listed above—and use your mantra, too. These little tips and tricks will really help you refresh, re-charge, and renew!

Wakeup time–noon: List your three essential morning activities, in order of priority, not including my morning stretch and meditation and breakfast. If you chose morning as the most likely time for personal time, add thirty minutes of personal time activity.

Now schedule your morning:

- *Morning stretch and meditation*
- *Breakfast* (at home or on the go)

_____

- *Me-time activity* (if you chose morning)

_____

Noon–5 PM: List your three essential afternoon activities, in order of priority, not including my afternoon stretch and lunch. If you chose afternoon as the most likely time for personal time, add thirty minutes of it.

Now schedule your afternoon:

- *Afternoon stretch* (once per hour if you have a desk job)
- *Lunch* (at home or on the go)

———————————————————————————————

- *Me-time activity* (if you chose afternoon)

———————————————————————————————

5 PM–bedtime: List your three essential evening activities, in order of priority, not including my bedtime stretch and dinner. If you chose evening as the most likely time for personal time, add thirty minutes of it.

Now schedule your evening:

- *Bedtime stretch*
- *Dinner* (at home or on the go)

———————————————————————————————

- *Me-time activity* (if you chose evening)

———————————————————————————————

Each week: Add one hour or more of personal time activity.

Every other weekend: Add one day or more of personal time activity.

CHAPTER 11

Get Energy Today! Your 14-Day PEP Plan

Welcome to your two-week personal energy plan! Armed with dozens of tips, techniques, and strategies designed to help you empower your body and love your life, you're ready to start living what you've learned so far. And I know you can do it!

For the next fourteen days, you'll focus on living in ways that increase your physical, mental, and emotional energy from morning till night. No more stressing through your mornings, yawning through your afternoons, or conking out on the couch after work, exhausted…this plan's got you covered, minute by minute. The best part: It's easy, it's quick, and it's fun!

First, I'll get your day off to a positive start with a daily dose of inspiration. (Someone dubbed these daily motivations "Deniseologies" a long time ago, and the name has stuck.) Each Deniseology addresses a different aspect of energy. Some days, we'll work on replenishing your physical energy; other days, we'll focus on your mental or emotional/spiritual energy.

Then simply follow the quick-and-easy morning, afternoon, and evening energy checklists, which all contain a tip or two to help you practice your daily "Deniseology." They're all small steps to try, but the idea is for you to continue to practice those tips that work for you.

Part of learning to live a healthier, more energetic lifestyle is to reflect on the changes you're making. The daily "Personal Energy Report" will help you keep track of your progress, and my morning and evening "Energy Questions" will help you begin and end each day with a positive attitude. Finally, I've given you ideas for energizing breakfasts and snacks, as well as a "break glass in case of emergency" tip for when you need a shot of energy, quick!

One last thing: No one knows you as well as you do, so feel free to tweak this plan in ways that fit your life. In fact, if you haven't done so already, why not fill out the Personal Energy Plan worksheet in chapter 10 before you begin this plan? It will help you see exactly where you can make positive changes that fit *your* schedule, habits, and lifestyle—changes that you may want to add to this plan. Then you've helped design a plan that's tailor-made for *you*!

DAY I

What kind of curve sets everything straight? A smile!

Start Energizing!

So many people tell me that they don't have time to exercise. The number one question I get is, "You're a mom, you work full-time...how do you find the time to work out?" My answer: Between my job and family, I never have time to exercise, either. I have to *make* the time!

As challenging as squeezing in that thirty-minute walk can be, it's your responsibility to make it happen. And if you do, the energy you'll gain will help you deal with every aspect of your life in a more positive, proactive way.

So when it comes to working out, don't let yourself off the hook. If you find yourself saying, "I don't have time to exercise," "I hate cardio!" or "I'm just too tired to work out," flip that negativity into positive action! How about "If I use the time I usually watch TV or surf the 'Net at night to exercise, I'll feel great tomorrow." Or "Cardio gets my blood moving, and energy begins with oxygen." Or "I'm tired because I sat on my butt all day. I may get to the gym tired, but I'll leave energized."

You know I'm right. Think about it: That sense of accomplishment as you end your workout is energizing in itself. And remember, you don't have to grind away on a treadmill for an hour—you only need thirty minutes of exercise every day to feel great!

In fact—skip the word *exercise* altogether. Try "I'm off to the gym to energize," or "I energize every morning before work." Sounds great, doesn't it? Before long, your body will catch up with your mind, and you'll look forward to "energizing." Even ten minutes a day is better than nothing. Just get moving!

Energy Emergency!

Soak up some sunlight. Get outside for ten minutes and turn your face to the sun! Research suggests that sunlight stimulates brain chemicals that improve mood. For an extra boost, get your sunlight first thing in the morning.

Morning Wake-Up Call

Down a cup of water.

Get up fifteen minutes early and take a brisk walk around your neighborhood.

Energizing breakfast: ½ whole-grain bagel with 1 tablespoon low-fat cream cheese, plus ½ cup berries or 1 orange.

Afternoon Pick-Me-Up

Do "perfect posture" body scans (see page 49).

Couldn't walk before work? Take that fifteen-minute walk during lunch!

Energizing snack: 1 small palmful almonds, plus ½ cup sliced fresh fruit or cut-up veggies with 1 tablespoon low-calorie dip of your choice.

After-Work and Evening Energy Boost

Do something outside when you get home from work for twenty minutes: garden or do yard work, play Frisbee with your kids or dog, or take your bike for a spin.

Refresh your spirit with some "me time."

TODAY'S PERSONAL ENERGY REPORT

When You Wake Up: Morning Energy Questions

- What will I look forward to today?
- What pleasure will I add to my day?
- How will I connect to someone today?

During the Day: Energy Checklist

☐ I got enough sleep last night.

☐ I energized with my morning stretch (see page 33).

☐ I ate breakfast.

☐ I drank eight glasses of water.

☐ I got outside for some fresh air and sunshine.

☐ I did my afternoon Energy Shot stretch (see page 37).

☐ If I caught myself slouching or slumping, I corrected my posture.

☐ If I caught myself in a negative thought, I turned it positive.

☐ I connected with someone.

☐ I did something fun or relaxing, just for me.

☐ I worked out for thirty minutes or more.

☐ I did my bedtime stretch (see page 42).

Before Bed: Evening Energy Questions

• Did I live the promises of my Morning Energy Questions?

• What fired me up today, and why?

• What tired me out today, and why?

DAY 2

Lift someone today, and let them lift you. That way, you'll both walk on air!

Appreciate the Most Affordable Luxury Today: Sleep!

Who doesn't like nice things? Soft, eight-hundred-thread-count sheets, ripe berries out of season, or a bouquet of fresh flowers on the kitchen table are treats that stimulate your senses and lift your spirits. Little luxuries like these are your reward for caring for the people who depend on you.

But there's one luxury that's totally free—eight solid, restful hours of sleep. Think about it: In this *go go go* world we live in, sleep is a luxury that few think they can afford. That's because time is at a premium, and in order to squeeze every last minute out of our day, we rob ourselves of our nightly opportunity to rest and recharge. And sometimes it's not chores that keep us up late, but stress. The day's work done, we then worry about the work that faces us tomorrow.

Why not treat yourself, each night, to a restful night's sle Remember when your kids were little, and you had a be ritual? First you bathed them, then fixed them a snack, t' them a bedtime story. Why not create your own ritual? An hour before bedtime, take a long, leisurely soak in a scented bath. Then fix yourself a cup of hot skim milk with a dash of vanilla and take up your knitting or read from a book of meditations. (No TV, no computer, and no mystery novels, which will stimulate rather than relax you.) Finally, slip into bed, tuck a cotton ball soaked in lavender oil under your pillow, put on your sleep mask, and slide into blissful slumber. In this frantic world, few things are more decadent than sleep. And this free "luxury" will guarantee you an energetic tomorrow!

Energy Emergency!

Treat your scalp to ninety seconds of bliss. A hairbrush massage stimulates nerve endings in the skin, which increases the brain's production of endorphins, University of Miami researchers found. The technique used in the study: Press the bristles of your hairbrush on your scalp. Stroke from your hairline to the base of your neck several times, then make small circles over your entire scalp. Alternate these methods for ninety seconds.

Morning Wake-Up Call
Wake up your senses and cleanse your liver by sipping a cup of
    hot water with a squeeze of lemon (I do every morning!).
Energizing breakfast: 1 cup high-fiber cereal with ¾ cup skim
    milk, plus ½ sliced banana or ½ cup berries.

Afternoon Pick-Me-Up
Take a fifteen-minute catnap if you need one. (No more than
    fifteen minutes, though!)
Energizing snack: 1 cup of air-popped popcorn.

After-Work and Evening Energy Boost

Take a thirty-minute walk several hours before bed to promote
restful sleep.

Take a long, warm soak before bed. If you like, add a few drops
of essential oil of lavender, long used to encourage a good
night's sleep.

TODAY'S PERSONAL ENERGY REPORT

When You Wake Up: Morning Energy Questions

- What will I look forward to today?
- What pleasure will I add to my day?
- How will I connect to someone today?

During the Day: Energy Checklist

- ☐ I got enough sleep last night.
- ☐ I energized with my morning stretch (see page 33).
- ☐ I ate breakfast.
- ☐ I drank eight glasses of water.
- ☐ I got outside for some fresh air and sunshine.
- ☐ I did my afternoon Energy Shot stretch (see page 37).
- ☐ If I caught myself slouching or slumping, I corrected my posture.
- ☐ If I caught myself in a negative thought, I turned it positive.
- ☐ I connected with someone.
- ☐ I did something fun or relaxing, just for me.
- ☐ I worked out for thirty minutes or more.
- ☐ I did my bedtime stretch (see page 42).

Before Bed: Evening Energy Questions

- Did I live the promises of my Morning Energy Questions?
- What fired me up today, and why?
- What tired me out today, and why?

DAY 3

Don't shy away from a challenge! Challenges make life interesting, and meeting them makes it meaningful.

Nourish Your Soul Today!

To nourish your body, you must eat healthy foods. But how do you nourish your soul? This is a worthwhile question, because if you feed your spirit a junk-food diet, your energy probably isn't what it could be.

The soul's equivalent of junk food is a life that lacks "nutrients" such as new experiences, joy, meaningful work and hobbies, and close relationships. If all you do is wake up, go to work, and come home again—and spend the moments in between doing chores, watching TV, or putting in laptop time—your soul doesn't get the nutrients it needs. In fact, it's starving! When you're starving, you reach for cookies and chips. When your soul is famished, you may buy things you don't need (and can't really afford), turn to food, cigarettes, or alcohol, or stay in friendships or relationships that deplete instead of feed your energy.

To nourish your soul, think about what makes you feel whole, alive, and one with the universe. While we are all unique, with different passions, some common sources of soul food include close and loving relationships, nature, art and music, meditation, walking, and prayer.

My most important sources of soul food are nature and time with my family and friends. I feed my soul when I cook and eat dinner with those closest to my heart, or walk along the beach when I'm in California. When I dip my toes in the waves or laugh with people I love, I feel rejuvenated—full of energy and connected to life.

To discover your soul food, tune into that soft voice within you. If you pause and listen, it will guide you to what you need. Once you discover those life-sustaining people, places, and things, nourish your soul with one or more of them every day!

Energy Emergency!

Call for backup. Ready to drop? Get some calming energy by calling the person who never fails to lift your spirits. As simple as this sounds, it works—but you've got to pick up the phone. Go on, dial her number, and let her positivity revive you!

Morning Wake-Up Call

Sip your coffee by the window with the best view, or enjoy it outside. Drink in the beauty (and quiet) of the morning.

Energizing breakfast: **Peanut Butter Cup Oatmeal:** 1 cup oatmeal mixed with ½ tablespoon natural peanut butter and 10 chocolate chips (optional); plus 1 piece string cheese.

Afternoon Pick-Me-Up

Look through the paper, or surf the web, to find a soul-nourishing activity for tonight or this weekend—a play, an antiques show, a concert, a local lecture or hike.

Energizing snack: 1 hard-boiled egg, 5 whole-grain crackers.

After-Work and Evening Energy Boost

If you found a soul-nourishing activity for this weekend, call a friend to invite her along.

Devote tonight to a hobby you've neglected. Knit, scrapbook, putter to your heart's content!

TODAY'S PERSONAL ENERGY REPORT

When You Wake Up: Morning Energy Questions

- What will I look forward to today?
- What pleasure will I add to my day?
- How will I connect to someone today?

During the Day: Energy Checklist

- ☐ I got enough sleep last night.
- ☐ I energized with my morning stretch (see page 33).
- ☐ I ate breakfast.
- ☐ I drank eight glasses of water.
- ☐ I got outside for some fresh air and sunshine.
- ☐ I did my afternoon Energy Shot stretch (see page 37).
- ☐ If I caught myself slouching or slumping, I corrected my posture.
- ☐ If I caught myself in a negative thought, I turned it positive.
- ☐ I connected with someone.
- ☐ I did something fun or relaxing, just for me.
- ☐ I worked out for thirty minutes or more.
- ☐ I did my bedtime stretch (see page 42).

Before Bed: Evening Energy Questions

- Did I live the promises of my Morning Energy Questions?
- What fired me up today, and why?
- What tired me out today, and why?

DAY 4

Love the moment, and the energy of that moment will spread beyond all boundaries. —Sister Mary Corita Kent

Having a Bad Day? Start Over!

Even optimists have what most people call "bad days." They spill mustard on their sweaters. Their umbrellas turn inside out in rainstorms. Their parking meters expire, and they get a ticket. I have the occasional bad day myself. (Just this morning, I had to clean up the mess my new puppy made on the carpet and call the plumber to fix a bad leak in my daughter's bathroom *and* my dishwasher!)

But I'll tell you a secret: Optimists' "bad days" are more like bad *moments*—and they brush them off like they would a crumb on their sleeve.

You know how sometimes you have a slice of cake, and you tell yourself you were "bad"? Well, a slice of cake isn't bad. It's a piece of cake. A bad day is simply a twenty-four-hour period that you've decided is defective. It's not the *day* that's bad—it's your *perception* of the day that stinks! But you can choose not to let a bad day own you—or steal your precious energy.

The next time you're in a bad mood that threatens to ruin your day, try this: Start your day over with a fresh attitude. Take a few deep breaths. Break for a cup of tea. Shrug your shoulders— literally—and say, "Oh, well." (Try it—it works!) Next, say the Serenity Prayer: "God grant me the serenity to accept the things I cannot change, the courage to change the things I can, and the wisdom to know the difference." Then pronounce your bad day through (even if it's still morning), and move on. When you choose to start your day over, you step outside the petty stuff and back into the big picture: Life is pretty darn good.

When you don't sweat the small stuff, you conserve mental and emotional energy that you can spend more wisely elsewhere. So if you're having a bad day, start it over with a more positive outlook—and resolve to make it better!

Energy Emergency!

Fight dinner-hour drowsiness with a song. Do you tend to get drowsy around dinnertime? Me too! It's because our bodies are exposed to the stress hormone cortisol all day, and our nervous systems are frazzled. To banish the dinner-hour drowsies, sing aloud for ten minutes. Melodic tones generate soothing vibrations in the brain that help reduce the output of cortisol.

Morning Wake-Up Call

Remind yourself to go with the flow today. Not sweating the small stuff conserves precious energy.

Energizing breakfast: **Cinnabagel:** Mix ¼ cup low-fat ricotta cheese, 1 teaspoon of jam, and a pinch of cinnamon; spread this on ½ whole-grain bagel, and enjoy with 1 apple or pear, sliced.

Afternoon Pick-Me-Up

In the chaos of the day, turn to your mantra or the Serenity Prayer. Repeat it, silently or out loud, until you feel positive and productive again.

Energizing snack: 1 high-protein bar.

After-Work and Evening Energy Boost

Sweat out a bad day on your cardio machine, or by doing my twenty-minute energy-boosting workout (chapter 12).

Need even more positivity? Rent your favorite comedy and
spend the night laughing.

TODAY'S PERSONAL ENERGY REPORT

When You Wake Up: Morning Energy Questions
- What will I look forward to today?
- What pleasure will I add to my day?
- How will I connect to someone today?

During the Day: Energy Checklist
- ☐ I got enough sleep last night.
- ☐ I energized with my morning stretch (see page 33).
- ☐ I ate breakfast.
- ☐ I drank eight glasses of water.
- ☐ I got outside for some fresh air and sunshine.
- ☐ I did my afternoon Energy Shot stretch (see page 37).
- ☐ If I caught myself slouching or slumping, I corrected my posture.
- ☐ If I caught myself in a negative thought, I turned it positive.
- ☐ I connected with someone.
- ☐ I did something fun or relaxing, just for me.
- ☐ I worked out for thirty minutes or more.
- ☐ I did my bedtime stretch (see page 42).

Before Bed: Evening Energy Questions
- Did I live the promises of my Morning Energy Questions?
- What fired me up today, and why?
- What tired me out today, and why?

DAY 5

When you follow your passion, you unleash your energy.
Let it flow like a river, and don't build any dams!

Make Over Your Morning Today!

How you begin your day usually sets the tone for the rest of your day. That's only natural—consistency and routine make it easier for us to do what we need to do. However, if you habitually hit the snooze button, a morning makeover can help you start every day with enthusiasm and energy.

Here's my morning ritual:

- Get up and do my morning stretch.
- Brush my teeth and make my bed.
- Pad to the kitchen for a glass of water with a squeeze of fresh lemon. My grandmother taught me this—the water rehydrates me, and the scent of fresh lemon stimulates my senses and wakes up my brain.
- Eat breakfast and savor family time—I may make the girls breakfast, or read the paper with my husband. And I always savor my *one* cup of coffee!
- Head to my home gym for my thirty-minute "energize" session.

Basically, I center myself and get into an organized and productive mind-set.

Your new morning ritual can be as short as five minutes or as long as fifteen. No matter how short it is, it will help you begin your day with so much more energy and enthusiasm.

As you do your makeover, think about how you might stimulate your senses in a gentle but positive way. Perhaps you could treat yourself to a highly fragrant tea, or your favorite coffee. Or you might keep a book of daily meditations by your bed and reach for it each morning, to frame the day ahead. Maybe a whimsical alarm clock would help you smile when you heard it, rather than groan? You don't have to spend a cent, though. Just pick two or three things that will add pleasure and reflection to your morning.

Oh, and pat yourself on the back. By giving your morning a redesign, you've set the stage for a positive, productive day!

Energy Emergency!

Get on your toes. Nodding off in a meeting? Excuse yourself, go to your office or the restroom, and bounce up and down on your toes. This will stimulate your circulatory system and deliver energizing oxygen to your cells. This works when you're drowsing on the couch after dinner, too.

Morning Wake-Up Call

If you don't have a morning ritual yet, spend a few minutes
    thinking about what you might do to make your morning
    more pleasant. How about reading for fifteen minutes before
    jumping in your car? Splurging on a favorite coffee? Asking
    your teenager to make his own breakfast? Then do it!
Energizing breakfast: Low-calorie breakfast sandwich with
    1 egg, 1 slice of turkey bacon, and a slice of low-fat cheese
    on half an English muffin, plus ¾ cup fresh blueberries.

Afternoon Pick-Me-Up

If you decided this morning how to remake your mornings,
    spend your lunch hour picking up any supplies you need—a
    book of morning meditations, that yummy coffee, easy and
    healthy breakfast foods for your kids, et cetera. (If you can't

get away, make a list, and pick them up on the way home
from work.)

Energizing snack: ½ cup cottage cheese with ½ cup berries or
other sliced fresh fruit.

After-Work and Evening Energy Boost

Spend a few minutes visualizing yourself waking up tomorrow
to your new morning ritual. The anticipation will lift your
spirits and boost your energy!

TODAY'S PERSONAL ENERGY REPORT

When You Wake Up: Morning Energy Questions

- What will I look forward to today?
- What pleasure will I add to my day?
- How will I connect to someone today?

During the Day: Energy Checklist

☐ I got enough sleep last night.

☐ I energized with my morning stretch (see page 33).

☐ I ate breakfast.

☐ I drank eight glasses of water.

☐ I got outside for some fresh air and sunshine.

☐ I did my afternoon Energy Shot stretch (see page 37).

☐ If I caught myself slouching or slumping, I corrected my posture.

☐ If I caught myself in a negative thought, I turned it positive.

☐ I connected with someone.

☐ I did something fun or relaxing, just for me.

☐ I worked out for thirty minutes or more.

☐ I did my bedtime stretch (see page 42).

Before Bed: Evening Energy Questions

- Did I live the promises of my Morning Energy Questions?
- What fired me up today, and why?
- What tired me out today, and why?

DAY 6

Attitude is everything—so pick a good one!

Lay Down Your Burden of Stress Today!

Stress is a burden you can't see, but you sure can feel it! Like any burden, if you carry it constantly, how much energy can you have? I heard this story years ago; it may help you put the burden of stress in perspective.

While giving a talk about stress management, the lecturer held up a glass of water. "How heavy is this glass of water?" he asked. A few members of the audience called out answers—eight ounces, ten ounces.

The lecturer replied, "What's important isn't its absolute weight, but how long you try to hold it. If I hold it for a minute, no problem. If I hold it for an hour, my arm will ache. If I hold it for a day, you'll have to call an ambulance. In each case, the glass is the same weight. But the longer I hold it, the heavier it becomes."

He continued, "That's the way it is with stress management. If we carry our burdens all the time, sooner or later, as the burden becomes heavier and heavier, we won't be able to carry it. As with this glass of water, you have to put it down for a while. When you're refreshed, you can pick it up again."

Never releasing the burden of stress harms the body and taxes the mind and spirit. So go ahead, put it down for a moment. Close your office door and do some deep breathing, go for a short v call a friend, pick up your knitting, or crank up your iPod and dance it out. These breaks really work if you use them—but to use them, you have to *choose* to bring peace and balance into your life.

What burden are you carrying at this moment? How long have you been carrying it? Whatever it is, put it down!

Energy Emergency!

Give fatigue the brush. Cleaning your teeth gives you a break, and that minty-fresh scent will pep you up. (I keep minty dental floss in my purse!) Keep a toothbrush at the office, and when you need a shot of energy, hit the ladies' room and brush with cinnamon-flavored or extra-minty toothpaste.

Morning Wake-Up Call

Ask yourself: *What do I need help with today?* Then ask someone—your partner, your mother, your best friend—to help you. Think of how much less stress you'd face if you knew you didn't have to come home to a load of laundry or go grocery shopping!

Energizing breakfast: Whole-grain English muffin spread with 2 tablespoons natural peanut butter, plus ½ cup sliced strawberries or melon.

Afternoon Pick-Me-Up

Need to blow off stress? Move it! Slip out for a quick stroll. Bounce up and down a flight of stairs once or twice. Do your afternoon stretch. To help you remember, set your watch alarm, or put a reminder on your computer's scheduling software.

Energizing snack: 1 ounce string cheese, plus 1 cup sliced fresh veggies (bell pepper, cucumber, carrots) with 2 tablespoons hummus.

After-Work and Evening Energy Boost

Yoga is a great way to relieve post-work stress. Dust off your yoga DVD and work your muscles while you calm your mind. Or drop in at a local class to see this de-stressing practice in action.

TODAY'S PERSONAL ENERGY REPORT

When You Wake Up: Morning Energy Questions

- What will I look forward to today?
- What pleasure will I add to my day?
- How will I connect to someone today?

During the Day: Energy Checklist

☐ I got enough sleep last night.

☐ I energized with my morning stretch (see page 33).

☐ I ate breakfast.

☐ I drank eight glasses of water.

☐ I got outside for some fresh air and sunshine.

☐ I did my afternoon Energy Shot stretch (see page 37).

☐ If I caught myself slouching or slumping, I corrected my posture.

☐ If I caught myself in a negative thought, I turned it positive.

☐ I connected with someone.

☐ I did something fun or relaxing, just for me.

☐ I worked out for thirty minutes or more.

☐ I did my bedtime stretch (see page 42).

Before Bed: Evening Energy Questions

• Did I live the promises of my Morning Energy Questions?
• What fired me up today, and why?
• What tired me out today, and why?

DAY 7

Enthusiasm breeds enthusiasm, and it is contagious. But whether you catch it or spread it, you will feel better. Be the most enthusiastic person you know today!

Use Your Energy Tool Kit Today!

Want to renew your vitality right now? You can if you want to. All you need to do is use one of the dozens of tips and techniques you've learned in this book. Each little suggestion is like a tool that can "fix" whatever is deflating your energy. Use the right tool, and you'll be right back on track!

Is your energy leak caused by negative thinking? The tool is thought-stopping. Identify your negative thought, then replace it with a positive one.

Is another person's negativity draining your enthusiasm? The tool is to excuse yourself. Even if it's just for five minutes. Shake off their negativity. If you can, find someone who exudes serenity, and soak it in.

Does your messy office dampen your motivation and productivity? The tool is a decluttering break. Clear your desk, and your mind will follow!

Are you depleted by the troubles of the world? You know what the tool is…turn that negative thought around! List three things that are going right in the world—people coming together for a common cause, for example.

Whatever drains your vitality, your energy tool kit contains a tool that you can use to neutralize it and move forward. If you live by this formula, you'll begin to see that there's rarely an excuse not to feel more energetic, immediately! (Sometimes, though, you just want to pout. Go on, indulge—but set a five-minute "pity party" limit.) Before long, you'll automatically pick the right tool for the job.

Energy Emergency!

Break for an emergency spa treatment. Weekday or weekend, slip into a scented bath, slather a mask on your face, and deep-condition your hair. If you can splurge, book an appointment at a day spa for a treatment you've always wanted to try—a hot-stone massage, for example. You deserve it!

Morning Wake-Up Call

Think about the tool that's given you the most energy over the past six days. What do you like about it? Why do you think it works for you? Resolve to use it today if you find that your energy is flagging.

Energizing breakfast: **Berry Nice Waffles:** Mix ½ cup low-fat cottage cheese, a dash of vanilla, and a dash of cinnamon; spoon over 2 low-fat waffles (fresh or from the freezer); top with ½ cup sliced berries.

Afternoon Pick-Me-Up

Dehydration can deplete your energy before you even feel thirsty. Is there a glass of water on your desk? If not, grab that empty glass and head for the water fountain!

Energizing snack: half an avocado with 1 warm corn tortilla or ½ cup berries or other sliced fresh fruit.

After-Work and Evening Energy Boost

Instead of falling on the couch and reaching for the remote, switch on your iPod. Listen to upbeat songs that really get your energy flowing. Dancing will get that energy flowing even more!

TODAY'S PERSONAL ENERGY REPORT

When You Wake Up: Morning Energy Questions

- What will I look forward to today?
- What pleasure will I add to my day?
- How will I connect to someone today?

During the Day: Energy Checklist

- ☐ I got enough sleep last night.
- ☐ I energized with my morning stretch (see page 33).
- ☐ I ate breakfast.
- ☐ I drank eight glasses of water.
- ☐ I got outside for some fresh air and sunshine.
- ☐ I did my afternoon Energy Shot stretch (see page 37).
- ☐ If I caught myself slouching or slumping, I corrected my posture.
- ☐ If I caught myself in a negative thought, I turned it positive.
- ☐ I connected with someone.
- ☐ I did something fun or relaxing, just for me.
- ☐ I worked out for thirty minutes or more.
- ☐ I did my bedtime stretch (see page 42).

Before Bed: Evening Energy Questions

- Did I live the promises of my Morning Energy Questions?
- What fired me up today, and why?
- What tired me out today, and why?

DAY 8

I still get wildly enthusiastic about little things...I play with leaves. I skip down the street and run against the wind. —Leo Buscaglia

Give Yourself Some Serenity Today!

When you hear the word *serenity*, what comes to mind? If you're like many people, serenity is a mysterious concept, a lofty state of mind open only to people who meditate in the lotus position or those in 12-step recovery groups. But you don't have to be a guru to achieve serenity. Believe me, serenity isn't mysterious. It's available to everyone, at any moment.

I define serenity as peace of mind, the feeling that all is well with you and your world. I feel serenity after I do a good workout, or when I'm with my family. You know you have serenity when your entire body relaxes and your heart seems to open. You won't necessarily feel happy, but you will feel settled, calm, and at peace.

Try this: Turn your mind to the issue that is most troubling to you at this moment. Feel that stress rise from your stomach to your chest? Feel your energy slipping away?

Now let go. Let that troubling situation just be. You don't have to fix it. All you have to do is acknowledge it, and then sit with it.

Think you can't? I know you can! Say the Serenity Prayer (page 181). Feel the power in those words? Carry them in your heart, repeat them whenever life gets crazy, and you'll connect with the truth in an instant: All is well!

> ### Energy Emergency!
>
> **Give yourself time off for good behavior.** No work, no chores, no errands. Take a day to do what *you* want to do. Sip cappuccino at your favorite bookstore. Browse your favorite junk stores. Take a day trip—as you roar down the highway, turn up the radio and sing along. Go on—you've earned it!

Morning Wake-Up Call

Before you get started on your day, take five minutes to meditate on a quotation that particularly inspires you, either from this book or from another source. Let its message seep into your mind, reminding you that all is well!

Energizing breakfast: **Toasted cheese sandwich:** Toast 2 slices whole-grain bread; top each slice with 1 slice low-fat cheese. Spread with mustard, if desired. Pop in the microwave for 15 seconds until the cheese melts. Serve with ½ cup grapes or 1 small apple.

Afternoon Pick-Me-Up

When stress and anxiety mount, use an old trick that really works: Count to ten, very slowly. As you count, stand up and stretch those muscles. Release their tension, and you'll calm your mind and spirit, too!

Energizing snack: ½ cup low-fat plain yogurt with ½ cup strawberries or 1 small banana.

After-Work and Evening Energy Boost

To find serenity tonight, turn to nature. You might take a walk, do some yard work, or watch the sun set. The beauty of nature can calm those jangling nerves and help you realize that however stressful your day has been, it's over and you can relax.

TODAY'S PERSONAL ENERGY REPORT

When You Wake Up: Morning Energy Questions
- What will I look forward to today?
- What pleasure will I add to my day?
- How will I connect to someone today?

During the Day: Energy Checklist
- ☐ I got enough sleep last night.
- ☐ I energized with my morning stretch (see page 33).
- ☐ I ate breakfast.
- ☐ I drank eight glasses of water.
- ☐ I got outside for some fresh air and sunshine.
- ☐ I did my afternoon Energy Shot stretch (see page 37).
- ☐ If I caught myself slouching or slumping, I corrected my posture.
- ☐ If I caught myself in a negative thought, I turned it positive.
- ☐ I connected with someone.
- ☐ I did something fun or relaxing, just for me.
- ☐ I worked out for thirty minutes or more.
- ☐ I did my bedtime stretch (see page 42).

Before Bed: Evening Energy Questions
- Did I live the promises of my Morning Energy Questions?
- What fired me up today, and why?
- What tired me out today, and why?

DAY 9

A smile on your face is like a light in your window: It tells people you're home.

Experience the Power of Wonder Today!

I'm a very curious person, especially about people. If I met you, chances are I'd ask where you were born, if you have kids, what you do, what you *like* to do, and a dozen other questions. My family and friends tease me sometimes about the way I ask people about themselves and their lives—they wonder if I'm conducting an interview! But that's just me. I love to see how people tick!

In fact, there are a lot of things in this world to wonder about—the world is a wonderful place! Or should I say, "wonder-full." There are miracles right under your nose! Suddenly you're *struck* by something you've seen or experienced countless times, and your soul taps into the rhythm of the universe. You notice the intricacy of a spider's web as you vacuum a dusty corner. A person very different from you touches your heart, and you realize that underneath we're all the same. You see a red bird in a green tree against a white winter sky, and you're awed by the beauty in the world.

Yet too many people live their lives believing that there is nothing new under the sun. How sad that would be if it were true!

Fortunately, it isn't. What *is* true, however, is that when you live a been-there-done-that life, day after day, you deflate your mental and emotional energy. Wonder is made up of equal parts curiosity, appreciation, and gratitude. Curiosity powers your mind; appreciation and gratitude, your spirit. Without a sense of wonder, there's little wonder that you'd go through life feeling lethargic and empty.

If that sounds like you, resolve to recapture the wonder that four-year-olds bring to every day, and that most adults misplace. Before long, you'll notice tiny surprises in every day. Your curiosity and creativity will be replenished.

Wonder grows wild everywhere, even in your own backyard. Put on your child-colored glasses and marvel at what you see. You might look out the kitchen door of your home, into your backyard at dusk. Suddenly a deer steps out of the tiny patch of woods on the edge of your property, then another. Don't you feel awed by their beauty? Doesn't it seem impossible that they're a part of the world you live in? But they are, and let that fact give you a quiet happiness.

Energy Emergency!

Awaken with grapefruit. Peel a grapefruit and breathe in the scent of the peel. Research has shown that the crisp aroma of this juicy citrus fruit can trigger an energizing jump in brain activity that can last for hours.

Morning Wake-Up Call

Spend the morning looking at the world with a four-year-old's eyes. Find things that excite your curiosity—a weather vane turning in the wind, an anthill in the crack of your walkway, a rainbow arcing across the sky after a rain shower. Stop to watch it for a minute or two, to marvel.

Energizing breakfast: 1 bowl of oatmeal with flaxseed and 1 cup berries.

Afternoon Pick-Me-Up

If you can, spend your lunch hour at the library (or stop in after work), and take out a book on a topic you've always found intriguing, but never had the time to ponder—astronomy, a fascinating personality from history, or the history of your favorite hobby. The world is a wondrous place—satisfy your curiosity about it!

Energizing snack: 1 hard-boiled egg on 1 slice whole-grain toast.

After-Work and Evening Energy Boost

If you can't remember the last time you experienced wonder, go to bed early tonight and then get up extra-early tomorrow to watch the sun come up. I'm serious—do it! I assure you, that been-there-done-that feeling will be replaced by awe and mystery. Let those feelings refill your spring of energy.

TODAY'S PERSONAL ENERGY REPORT

When You Wake Up: Morning Energy Questions

- What will I look forward to today?
- What pleasure will I add to my day?
- How will I connect to someone today?

During the Day: Energy Checklist

- ☐ I got enough sleep last night.
- ☐ I energized with my morning stretch (see page 33).
- ☐ I ate breakfast.
- ☐ I drank eight glasses of water.
- ☐ I got outside for some fresh air and sunshine.
- ☐ I did my afternoon Energy Shot stretch (see page 37).

☐ If I caught myself slouching or slumping, I corrected my posture.

☐ If I caught myself in a negative thought, I turned it positive.

☐ I connected with someone.

☐ I did something fun or relaxing, just for me.

☐ I worked out for thirty minutes or more.

☐ I did my bedtime stretch (see page 42).

Before Bed: Evening Energy Questions

• Did I live the promises of my Morning Energy Questions?

• What fired me up today, and why?

• What tired me out today, and why?

DAY 10

Energy isn't just about how fast your feet move. It's also about how open your heart is. Power your mind with positive thoughts, put a smile on your face, and you're halfway there!

Take the "Boredom Challenge" Today!

Sure, you're busy. You've got a family to care for, a job, and a to-do list a mile long. Your days are full, but your life seems stale and predictable. You're just going through the motions. You're restless and irritable. You're bored.

Boredom is a sign of unutilized potential. It's also a passive state, and a passive state is a low-energy state. But here's the positive side of boredom: It's a call to action from your soul, telling you that you need to test your boundaries.

If you're plagued by chronic boredom, the only one who can relieve you is *you*! It's your responsibility to harness all that mental and creative force into an activity that engages and stimulates you. The challenge is to identify what that activity might be. Maybe you want to write a novel or start a daily blog. How about pursuing a spiritual practice, such as prayer or meditation? You could find a new way to move your body through dance or yoga, or learn a martial art like tai chi or karate. Maybe you want to master a specific craft, such as making soap or throwing pottery. The possibilities are endless—and they're all up to you!

While boredom can be painful, it can also be the trigger for personal growth. It can give you the opportunity to stretch yourself, go beyond your boundaries, and that's always a good thing. When you answer its call, that restlessness will be replaced by enthusiasm and boundless creative energy!

Energy Emergency!

Redo your to-do list. Do you need to wrangle with your cell phone provider or deal with some other pesky situation? Get it done, then reward yourself with a small treat, like twenty minutes at the mall or on a park bench. When you can cross that task off your list, you'll be amazed by the rush of energy you feel.

Morning Wake-Up Call

Think about one activity you would be willing to pursue thirty to sixty minutes a day, every day. Whatever it is, it should stimulate your mind, tap into your creativity, and engage your soul. Then take steps to make it happen. Sign up for a website that allows you to research your family tree. Juggle your schedule to fit in that one-hour walk, then put it on your to-do list. Institute a one-hour "library time," where you sit down and do nothing but read. Even preparing to do it will ease your boredom!

Energizing breakfast: ½ whole-grain bagel with 1 tablespoon low-fat cream cheese, served with ½ cup berries or 1 orange.

Afternoon Pick-Me-Up

Spend a few minutes researching the activity you picked this morning. Make the e-mails or calls necessary to set the wheels in motion—surf genealogy groups to select one, call a sibling or friend to ask if she wants to walk with you, make a list of five books you want to read or research local book-discussion groups in your area.

Energizing snack: 1 piece string cheese, plus ½ cup berries or other sliced fresh fruit.

After-Work and Evening Energy Boost

Puzzle yourself this evening! Do a crossword, sudoku, or other brain teaser to exercise your mind. Or simply continue to set up your plans for the activity you selected this morning.

TODAY'S PERSONAL ENERGY REPORT

When You Wake Up: Morning Energy Questions
- What will I look forward to today?
- What pleasure will I add to my day?
- How will I connect to someone today?

During the Day: Energy Checklist
- ☐ I got enough sleep last night.
- ☐ I energized with my morning stretch (see page 33).
- ☐ I ate breakfast.
- ☐ I drank eight glasses of water.
- ☐ I got outside for some fresh air and sunshine.

☐ I did my afternoon Energy Shot stretch (see page 37).

☐ If I caught myself slouching or slumping, I corrected my posture.

☐ If I caught myself in a negative thought, I turned it positive.

☐ I connected with someone.

☐ I did something fun or relaxing, just for me.

☐ I worked out for thirty minutes or more.

☐ I did my bedtime stretch (see page 42).

Before Bed: Evening Energy Questions

• Did I live the promises of my Morning Energy Questions?

• What fired me up today, and why?

• What tired me out today, and why?

DAY 11

Loan a smile to someone who needs one. They'll repay it—with interest!

Get Over Carb Phobia Today!

Do you feel guilty if you eat a big plate of pasta or a serving of rice because it contains "too many carbs"? Let me tell you something. If carbs caused weight gain, I would be in trouble, because I love my fruit, grains, and bread!

Here's the scientific truth: Your body needs carbs. They are its preferred source of energy. If you severely restrict them, you'll have as much energy as a wet noodle. You'll drag yourself through your days, feel mentally exhausted, and certainly won't have the energy to work out.

Now, it's true that when it comes to carbohydrates, portions count. If you eat one serving of pasta—about a cup—you'll be fine. Four or five servings? Not so much. I cringe when I'm in a restaurant and see a waiter serve pasta on a plate the size of a hubcap!

The *kind* of carbs you select counts, too. While it's fine to enjoy doughnuts, ice cream, and other simple carbohydrates as an occasional treat, a steady diet of them will plump you up.

Foods high in white sugar and flour also deflate your energy. That's because their sugars enter your bloodstream rapidly. In an attempt to move all that sugar out of the blood, the levels of insulin in your blood spike. A short time later, insulin has done its job, and your blood sugar crashes. Unfortunately, so do you!

If you eat mostly complex carbs—fruit, veggies, beans, and whole grains—and pay attention to portion sizes, you won't gain weight. What you *will* gain: energy! Complex carbs are packed with nutrients. They're also rich in fiber, which helps keep your blood sugar on an even keel, so your body and brain receive a steady supply of energy. Fiber also keeps you fuller, longer, meaning you are less likely to overeat—and more likely to feel energetic!

Energy Emergency!

Give yourself a minty wake-up call. Add a few drops of peppermint essential oil to a large bowl of cool water. Dip a clean washcloth in the bowl, wring it out, and place the cloth over your face. Inhale deeply. The fresh, minty scent will clear your head instantly!

Morning Wake-Up Call

Whip up the healthy breakfast smoothie below, made with sweet, creamy banana and vanilla almond milk. Almond milk is made from almonds and filtered water, along with vanilla flavoring. It has all the nutrients of milk, and contains just ninety calories per cup. (You can use regular low-fat milk, too, if you like.) It's quick, easy, and simply delicious!

Energizing breakfast: **Banana-Vanilla Almond Milk Smoothie**
   1 cup vanilla-flavored almond milk or 1 cup low-fat milk
   1 small banana, sliced
   Dash of vanilla extract
   2–3 ice cubes
Place all the ingredients in your blender. Blend, pour, and enjoy!

Afternoon Pick-Me-Up

Today, or tonight after work, stop at the grocery store and
   fill your basket with healthy carbs such as brown rice or
   quinoa—a seed with a nutty taste and fluffy texture, usually
   stocked in the organic aisles. Pick up some crunchy salad
   greens, sweet berries, and brightly colored bell peppers, too.
   Make these and other healthy carbs the foundation of all
   your meals and you'll take a big step toward more energy
   and better health!
Energizing snack: 2 tablespoons hummus, spread on 1 whole-
   grain rice cake or dip into it with carrots and celery.

After-Work and Evening Energy Boost

Treat yourself to a serving of brown rice at dinner tonight, or
   enjoy an English muffin for breakfast. They'll give your
   body the fuel it needs without widening your waistline!

TODAY'S PERSONAL ENERGY REPORT

When You Wake Up: Morning Energy Questions

- What will I look forward to today?
- What pleasure will I add to my day?
- How will I connect to someone today?

During the Day: Energy Checklist

☐ I got enough sleep last night.

☐ I energized with my morning stretch (see page 33).

☐ I ate breakfast.

☐ I drank eight glasses of water.

☐ I got outside for some fresh air and sunshine.

☐ I did my afternoon Energy Shot stretch (see page 37).

☐ If I caught myself slouching or slumping, I corrected my posture.

☐ If I caught myself in a negative thought, I turned it positive.

☐ I connected with someone.

☐ I did something fun or relaxing, just for me.

☐ I worked out for thirty minutes or more.

☐ I did my bedtime stretch (see page 42).

Before Bed: Evening Energy Questions

• Did I live the promises of my Morning Energy Questions?

• What fired me up today, and why?

• What tired me out today, and why?

DAY 12

If you have built castles in the air, your work need not be lost; that is where they should be. Now put foundations under them. —Henry David Thoreau

Fake It Till You Make It Today!

More than a century ago, American psychologist William James taught, "If you want a quality, act as if you already have it." From this insight, the expression "Fake it until you make it"—sometimes called "Act as if"—was born. The idea is to fake positive behaviors, particularly confidence and enthusiasm, until you really feel them. You might think of this technique as a dress rehearsal for succ

Because energy flows from positivity, try "faking" energizing behaviors until they become second nature. Here's an easy way to do it: Think of the most high-energy person you know. Then analyze this person from head to toe. What do you see that makes her so vibrant, so positive?

You might first notice that she stands straight, looks into your eyes when she talks to you, and perhaps even puts her hand on your arm. She probably has a sparkle in her eyes and an open, friendly smile, too. What you can *feel*, but not see, is that she inspires others to do, and be, their best. She believes in you so strongly, you can't help but believe in yourself.

Once you've identified her high-energy traits, steal them! (Remember: Imitation is the sincerest form of flattery.) Copy how she walks, talks, and acts—and try, even, to copy how she thinks. If you continue to act as if you are an upbeat, high-energy person, you will soon become one.

There's no doubt that what we do, habitually, affects how we feel. William James said it best: "We don't laugh because we're happy—we're happy because we laugh."

So the next time you want to pull the covers over your head in the morning, think of your vivacious role model one second before her alarm clock sounds. She opens her eyes. What does she do next? Whatever it is, do the same!

Energy Emergency!

Step it up! When the midafternoon slump hits, don't hit the vending machine. Instead go up and down a flight of steps, twice, to boost your circulation and deliver fresh oxygen to your muscles and brain.

Morning Wake-Up Call

Take a calculated risk in your personal life or at work. I don't
   mean something dangerous, but something that makes you
   feel *alive*—standing up for something that's important to you,
   or doing something you want to do but aren't sure you can.
   Your risk may or may not pay off, but when you step outside
   your comfort zone, you can't help but feel more fired up!

Energizing breakfast: 1 cup high-fiber cereal with ¾ cup skim
   milk, plus ½ sliced banana or ½ cup berries.

Afternoon Pick-Me-Up

Decide on a personality trait you'd like to acquire, and then
   take one action a week for the next four weeks to help you
   acquire that trait. For example, say you'd like to become
   more outgoing. This week, start with a simple action, such
   as asking a stranger for directions. Next week, you might
   introduce yourself to the head of the PTA and tell her that
   great new fund-raising idea you have. Before you know it,
   you'll have acquired several new ways to be outgoing, and
   you can build on them until you're no longer faking it!

Energizing snack: 5 whole-grain crackers spread with 1 tablespoon natural peanut butter and 2 teaspoons jelly.

After-Work and Evening Energy Boost

List one thing you've always wanted to do, but haven't. Suppose
   you've always wanted to act in community theater, but have
   made excuses as to why you can't (too shy, can't sing or
   dance, you'd forget your lines, and so forth). Write down
   every reason you *can't*, and then demolish each excuse. Next,
   set a goal to go to an audition within the next three months.
   You can do anything you set your mind to—remember, you
   always have choices!

TODAY'S PERSONAL ENERGY REPORT

When You Wake Up: Morning Energy Questions

- What will I look forward to today?
- What pleasure will I add to my day?
- How will I connect to someone today?

During the Day: Energy Checklist

- ☐ I got enough sleep last night.
- ☐ I energized with my morning stretch (see page 33).
- ☐ I ate breakfast.
- ☐ I drank eight glasses of water.
- ☐ I got outside for some fresh air and sunshine.
- ☐ I did my afternoon Energy Shot stretch (see page 37).
- ☐ If I caught myself slouching or slumping, I corrected my posture.
- ☐ If I caught myself in a negative thought, I turned it positive.
- ☐ I connected with someone.
- ☐ I did something fun or relaxing, just for me.
- ☐ I worked out for thirty minutes or more.
- ☐ I did my bedtime stretch (see page 42).

Before Bed: Evening Energy Questions

- Did I live the promises of my Morning Energy Questions?
- What fired me up today, and why?
- What tired me out today, and why?

DAY 13

Your imagination is your preview of life's coming attractions. —Albert Einstein

Celebrate the Miracle of You Today!

No matter how busy you are, chances are that each year, on your birthday, you pamper yourself without apology. You sleep in, take the day off, or go out to lunch or dinner. You bask in the well wishes of family, friends, and co-workers, and thoroughly enjoy the fuss made over you. It's a day that's all for you—no one expects you to do the dishes or the laundry, and you might even get breakfast in bed!

What if you could live a small part of each day as if it were your birthday? You could, for example, celebrate the "gifts" you've received that day, such as a compliment at work, a smile from a stranger, a good deed done for you alone, or a spot of serenity in an otherwise crazy day. You could pamper yourself in one small way each day, as you do on your birthday. For example, you might sneak out of work half an hour early on a beautiful day, treat yourself to a pedicure, or take an hour for yourself and work on your scrapbook, or go to a movie you want to see in blissful solitude.

Each day, in some small way, you could celebrate your life and who you are. You are unique—there is no one quite like you in the entire world. It's a miracle that you're here, and there are more miracles to come, because when you live with positivity and gratitude, each and every day is filled with wonder, joy, and love.

Every day, you can be reborn. Every day, you can give thanks for the ultimate gift: another day of life. Happy birthday!

> ### Energy Emergency!
>
> **Give your ears a rubdown.** Wrapped in a mental fog? In Chinese medicine, when you stimulate your ears, you redirect your energy upward to your head. So show those earlobes some love—gently, of course!

Morning Wake-Up Call

Let yourself sparkle a bit today. Spritz yourself with your favorite perfume—the one that you usually save for special occasions. (*You're* the occasion today!) Wear your best lingerie set under your jeans and T-shirt or work clothes. Pull your hair back with a pretty comb or barrette, and wear lipstick and mascara.

Energizing breakfast: Low-calorie breakfast sandwich—I make mine open-faced with 1 scrambled egg and 1 piece of turkey bacon on half an English muffin, and sometimes a touch of low-fat cheese, plus 1 small whole apple, orange, or pear.

Afternoon Pick-Me-Up

Remember when your mom used to put your drawings on the refrigerator with a magnet? It felt good, didn't it? Well, you can recapture that feeling of pride and accomplishment. Jot down three things you've recently accomplished and feel good about. Maybe you lost five pounds, baked the perfect loaf of bread, and got to the gym every day last week. Then, from that list, pick one to proudly tell to someone who loves and supports you—your partner, kids, a special co-worker, a parent or best friend. Bask in their praise—you've earned it!

Energizing snack: 1 mini bag microwave popcorn and 1 piece string cheese.

After-Work and Evening Energy Boost

What three things do you love most about yourself? Don't be bashful—it's time to toot your own horn a bit! You are a unique individual with special talents, and it's time to unleash them on the world! A good way to begin is to ask yourself, each day, *What can I do today to develop my gifts and give more of myself to others?*

TODAY'S PERSONAL ENERGY REPORT

When You Wake Up: Morning Energy Questions
- What will I look forward to today?
- What pleasure will I add to my day?
- How will I connect to someone today?

During the Day: Energy Checklist
- ☐ I got enough sleep last night.
- ☐ I energized with my morning stretch (see page 33).
- ☐ I ate breakfast.
- ☐ I drank eight glasses of water.
- ☐ I got outside for some fresh air and sunshine.
- ☐ I did my afternoon Energy Shot stretch (see page 37).
- ☐ If I caught myself slouching or slumping, I corrected my posture.
- ☐ If I caught myself in a negative thought, I turned it positive.
- ☐ I connected with someone.
- ☐ I did something fun or relaxing, just for me.
- ☐ I worked out for thirty minutes or more.
- ☐ I did my bedtime stretch (see page 42).

Before Bed: Evening Energy Questions

- Did I live the promises of my Morning Energy Questions?
- What fired me up today, and why?
- What tired me out today, and why?

DAY 14

Let a joy keep you. Reach out your hands and take it when it runs by. —*Carl Sandburg*

Reflect on How Far You've Come!

Congratulations—you've come to the end of this program, but you've just begun what is hopefully a life of new vitality, zest, and joy. You've learned a lot on the first leg of this journey, and you're ready to fly solo.

As you continue the process of becoming a more positive, energetic you, keep in mind that there is more to this process than changing your thinking and attitude. Just as you can gauge your weight loss by stepping on a scale regularly, you can, and should, measure your progress another way—by taking stock of how you feel. Is your energy level increasing? Are you nipping negative thoughts in the bud, and getting enough sleep? These are important signs of growth and change—and by paying attention to them, you'll be doing yourself a big favor!

Remember that a strong component of a more energetic lifestyle is reflection—taking your own pulse so you can begin to notice what tires you out and what fires you up, what works for you and what doesn't. Be alert to changes in your energy level, your mood, your connections with others, how quickly you fall asleep at night, and how rested you feel in the morning. Above all, be honest with yourself about your high and low moments. One of the most exciting and rewarding moments in your personal journey to a more vibrant life is to reflect back and realize how much you've changed. Be proud of yourself for how far you've come!

Energy Emergency!

Lock yourself in the ladies' room. Or your own bathroom. Focus on one object—say, your shower curtain—and do the "observe and report" that is mindfulness meditation (the technique is discussed on pages 86–87). Feel your mind clear and your serenity return.

Morning Wake-Up Call

Because positive thinking is so important to all-day energy, it can't hurt to have some instant positive reinforcement on hand! On an index card, write down two or more inspiring quotations to say silently or out loud, then tuck the card in your wallet. When negative thinking or the blues strike, take out your card, say your affirmations, and sweep them away!

Energizing breakfast: **Berry Good Sundae**

8 ounces low-fat fruit yogurt

⅛ teaspoon vanilla

¼ teaspoon cinnamon

¾ cup low-sugar, high-fiber cereal

½ cup berries, washed and sliced

In a small bowl, combine the yogurt, vanilla, and cinnamon. Spoon a dollop of the yogurt mixture into a parfait glass, a champagne flute, or a small wineglass with a narrow bowl. Top with cereal; then add a layer of berries. Alternate layers until the glass is full.

Afternoon Pick-Me-Up

Think of a positive affirmation that helps you honor your commitment to an energizing lifestyle, and then make it your
computer's new screen saver. One affirmation might be, "I
choose to live in ways that energize and uplift me," but the
best one will come not from me, but from your heart!
Change them whenever you need a shot of motivation and
to recommit to your new, energetic lifestyle. It's a great way
to remind yourself to take care of your body, have a positive
attitude, and do the things you *know* give you energy!

Energizing snack: 1 small palmful almonds, served with ½ cup
sliced fresh fruit or cut-up veggies with 1 tablespoon
low-calorie dip of your choice.

After-Work and Evening Energy Boost

Choose a photo of yourself as a child where you're in action—
swinging on a swing, jumping off a diving board, smiling as
you ride your bike or romp with your dog. Frame it, then
place it somewhere you'll see it every day—perhaps on your
nightstand next to your alarm clock, or on your kitchen
windowsill. Every time you see it, let that image of pure
energy reconnect you with that vital, passionate part of
yourself. You still have that fire within you, and you can
keep it burning for as long as you live!

TODAY'S PERSONAL ENERGY REPORT

When You Wake Up: Morning Energy Questions

- What will I look forward to today?
- What pleasure will I add to my day?
- How will I connect to someone today?

During the Day: Energy Checklist

☐ I got enough sleep last night.

☐ I energized with my morning stretch (see page 33).

☐ I ate breakfast.

☐ I drank eight glasses of water.

☐ I got outside for some fresh air and sunshine.

☐ I did my afternoon Energy Shot stretch (see page 37).

☐ If I caught myself slouching or slumping, I corrected my posture.

☐ If I caught myself in a negative thought, I turned it positive.

☐ I connected with someone.

☐ I did something fun or relaxing, just for me.

☐ I worked out for thirty minutes or more.

☐ I did my bedtime stretch (see page 42).

Before Bed: Evening Energy Questions

• Did I live the promises of my Morning Energy Questions?

• What fired me up today, and why?

• What tired me out today, and why?

CHAPTER 12

Your 20-Minute Energy-Boosting, Muscle-Firming Workout

Get ready to firm and tone up your body and pump up your energy with this all-new workout!

I divided the routine into four mini circuits of five minutes each. *The cardio workout* gives you instant energy by getting your blood moving and that oxygen flowing. *The toning routine* combines yoga and light weights, two of my favorite ways to sculpt and tone your muscles from head to toe. You can use a set of three-, five-, or eight-pound dumbbells—choose what's best for you. *The ab/core workout* zeros in on your abs and core to flatten your tummy and trim your waist. *The power/balance routine* consists of "power moves" that improve your balance and infuse you with that great calm energy.

Best of all, you only have to do each exercise for one minute. But do the entire routine faithfully, and the results can last a lifetime. To thrive longer...get stronger!

You can also mix and match these five-minute routines to suit your needs or schedule. If you're pressed for time or need a quick burst of energy, do one or two of the routines of your choice. If you have twenty minutes, do all four. Do the full routine every day if you can—you'll see great results sooner than you think!

Perform each of these twenty moves for one minute each.

For Instant Energy: 5-Minute Cardio Blast

Jump Start for Energy

Jump to it! This move revs up both your metabolism and your energy.

A. Stand tall with your legs together and your arms by your sides.

B. Jump out and forward about a foot and land softly in a squat, with your knees bent and feet wider than hip-width apart. Try to sit back with your weight through your heels. See if you can touch your elbows to your thighs. Then jump back with your feet together to the starting position. Keep jumping out and in, forward and back.

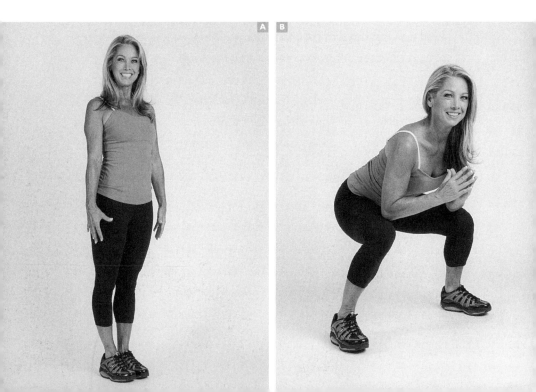

Front Kick/Lunge Back

This exercise stimulates your muscle tone and blood circulation to infuse you with energy.

A. Stand tall and kick your right leg out in front of you (straighten the leg without locking your knees). Reach your left arm toward your right leg. Tighten your abs.

B. Then lunge your right leg back straight behind you as you bend your left knee and place your left hand on your left thigh for balance. Do this for 30 seconds, then switch legs and repeat.

C. For an extra challenge, touch your fingertips to the floor on your lunges.

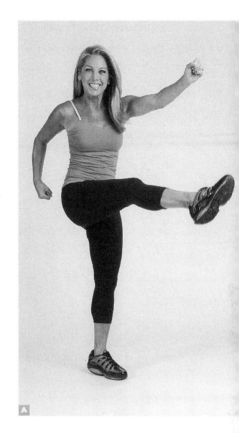

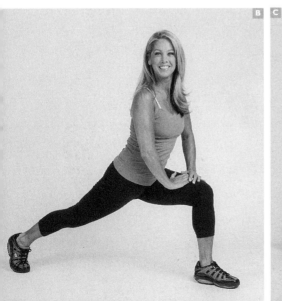

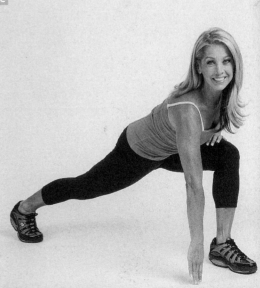

Football Drill/Quick Feet

This move helps pump oxygen to every cell in the body!

Stand tall with your feet wider than hip-width apart. Bend your knees as you sit back into a wide squat stance. Bend your arms in front of your chest as if you're holding a small ball. Raise your right foot (about an inch) and bring your right knee up from the floor. Then lower your right foot and repeat with your left foot. Alternate feet as quickly as you can, keeping your abs tight and your back strong.

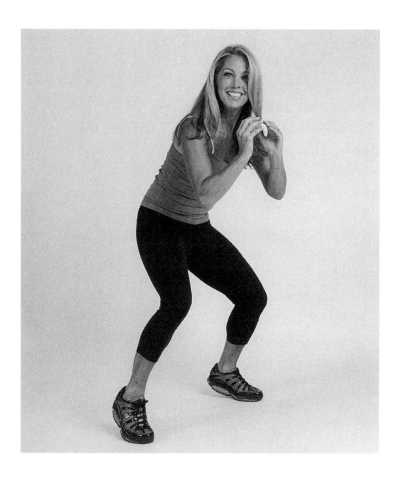

Ski Jumps

Energize with plyometrics, a great way to blast fat and pump up your energy!

Stand tall with your feet together and your arms by your sides.

A. Sit back into a squat to the right side, keeping your back straight and your abs pulled in.
B. From the side ski squat, jump into the air using your arms.
C. As you land to the left side, bend your knees softly to minimize impact. Continue to jump from side to side.

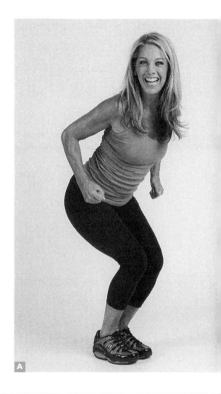

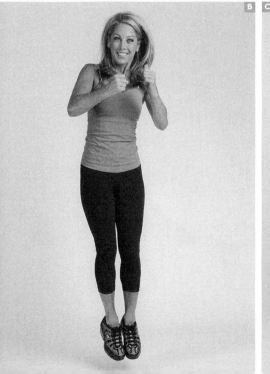

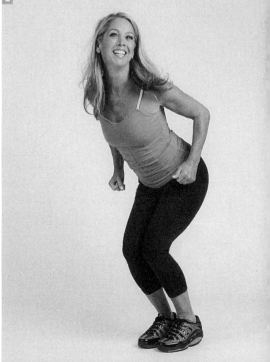

Mountain Climbers

This total-body exercise will help your energy soar straight to the top!

A. Begin in plank position (like a push-up), balancing on your hands and your toes. Keep your back straight and your abs pulled in. Your body should form one long line from the top of your head to your heels.

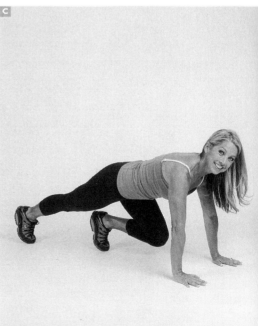

B. Quickly bring your right knee forward, then quickly straighten it out behind you.

C. Repeat with your left knee. Keep pumping, with your knees alternating as quickly as you can.

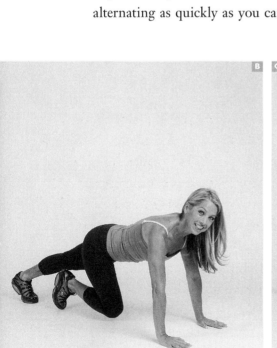

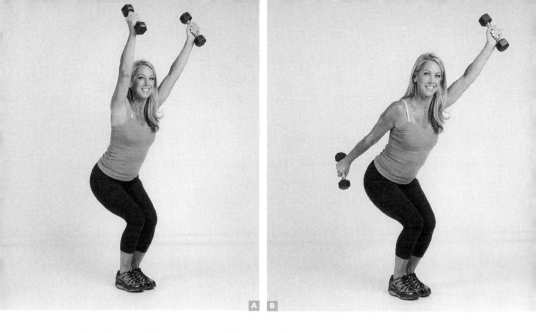

A B

To Firm Up Fast: 5-Minute Toning Workout

These exercises, which combine yoga with light weights, are designed to firm and tone you from head to toe. You'll need three-, five-, or eight-pound dumbbells, depending on your strength.

Chair Squat with Front Raises
This combination exercise sculpts beautiful shoulders and streamlines your legs.

A. Stand with your feet together holding your dumbbells in front of your thighs, with your palms facing your thighs. Draw your navel in toward your spine and roll your shoulders down your back to set your posture. Bend your knees, aiming for ninety degrees, squeezing your inner thighs together. Keeping your core engaged the entire time, lift your arms over your head with your biceps by your ears, maintaining a long spine.

B. With your left arm still extended, lower your right arm, reaching it behind you. Bring your right arm up and over your head as you lower your left arm. Repeat, alternating right and left, keeping your back lengthened and your legs and core fully engaged.

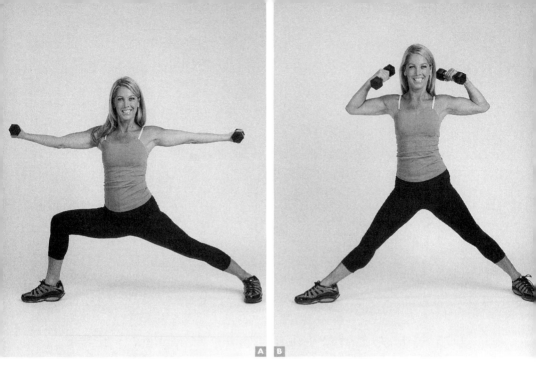

A **B**

Warrior with Bicep Curls
This combo move firms your arms and thighs.

A. Stand with your feet shoulder-width apart, your arms at your sides, and the dumbbells in your hands. With your right foot, step out to the right side about three feet. Turn your right foot out at a forty-five-degree angle and—keeping your left leg straight—bend your right leg so that it is directly in line with your ankle, forming a ninety-degree angle. Lower yourself into a lunge. Once your foundation is set in Warrior, lift your arms out to the sides at shoulder height, rotating in the shoulder socket so that your palms are facing up.

B. Inhale to root yourself into the ground with strong legs and exhale as you slowly curl your hands toward your shoulders, keeping your upper arms parallel to the floor at the same time as you straighten your right leg. Inhale as you extend your arms and bend your right knee again. Repeat for 30 seconds, then switch legs.

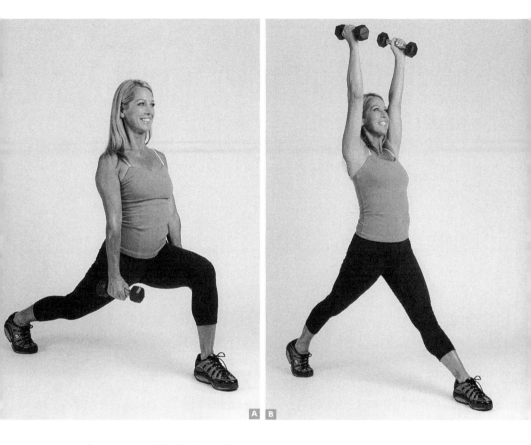

A B

Crescent with Triceps Toners

This dynamic move tones your thighs as it firms the back of your arms.

A. Stand nice and tall, with your hands at your sides and the dumbbells in your hands facing in toward your body. Take a large step back with your right leg and bend your left knee, making sure it is at a ninety-degree angle and your feet are shoulder-width apart.

B. Exhale as you push into your front (left) foot and straighten both legs while at the same time extending your arms over your head.

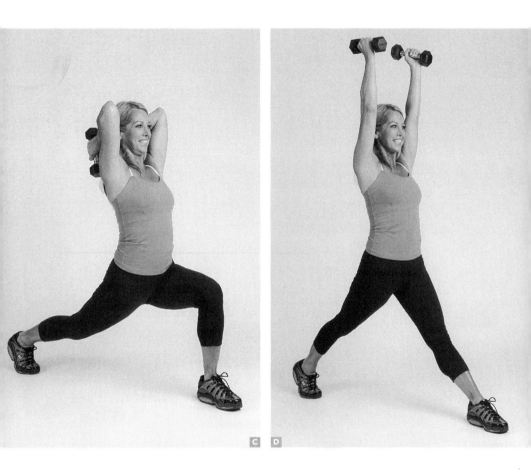

C. Bend your elbows to lower the dumbbells until they are behind your shoulders and your elbows are pointing toward the ceiling as you bend your left leg and lunge.

D. Straighten your front leg and extend your arms overhead. Repeat for 30 seconds, then switch to the other leg.

Side Angle with Rows

Trim your waistline and sculpt your back with one simple exercise.

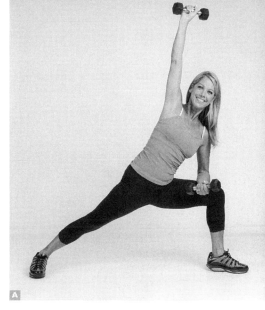

A. Stand with your feet shoulder-width apart, your arms at your sides, and the dumbbells in your hands. With your left foot, step out to the left side about three feet. Turn your left foot out at a forty-five-degree angle and—keeping your right leg straight—bend your left leg so that it is directly in line with your ankle, forming a ninety-degree angle. Lower yourself into a lunge. Place your left elbow on your left thigh and raise your right arm up to the ceiling.

B. Slowly lower your right arm toward the floor.

C. Draw your right elbow up to row and continue to reach your right arm back up to the ceiling. Repeat for 30 seconds, then switch sides.

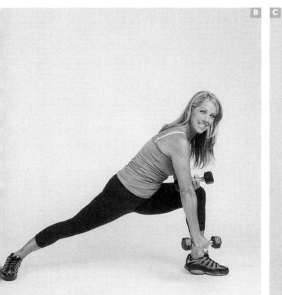

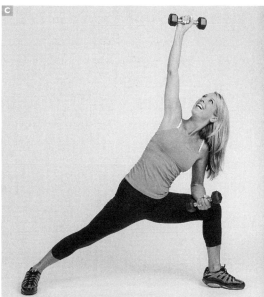

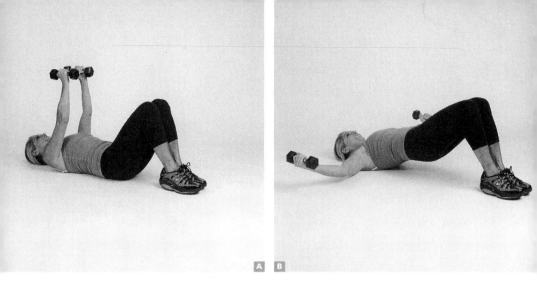

A B

Bridge with Chest Flies

This powerful combo move lifts your tush and chest.

A. Lie on your back with your knees bent and your feet flat on the floor. Hold the dumbbells above your chest with your arms slightly bent.

B. Inhale and slowly pull your arms out to either side. Engage your chest muscles and bring your arms back over your chest as you squeeze your glutes to lift your hips off the floor. Pull your navel to your spine and try to squeeze your inner thighs together for a more intense core workout. Repeat for 1 minute.

C. For an extra challenge: Lift one leg when your hips are off the mat.

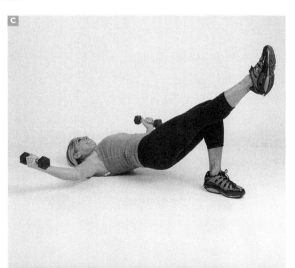

To Tone Your Tummy: 5-Minute Ab and Core Workout

This is an awesome tummy-tightening routine! Make sure you have a tea towel for resistance and assistance, which will help prevent neck strain and improve your alignment.

Ab and Back Strengthener
This exercise articulates the spine in both directions, extension and flexion.

A. Sit up tall with your knees bent and your feet flat on the floor. Place the towel under your thighs, and hold both ends taut.

B. Inhale as you pull your shoulders down and back, then exhale as you contract your abs and round your low back to hollow out through the tummy. Repeat for 1 minute.

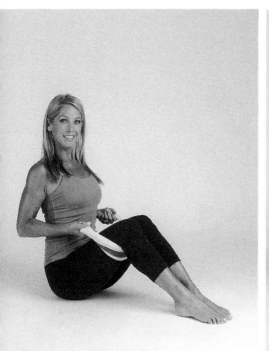
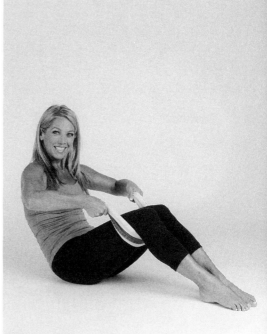

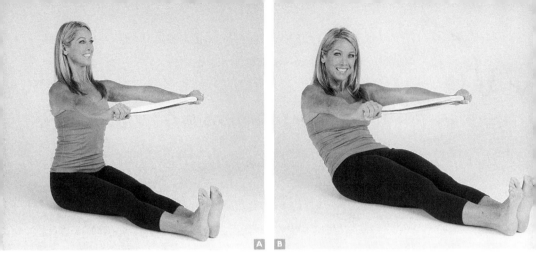

For an extra challenge, add the Roll Down:

A. Sit tall, back straight, chest lifted, with your legs straight out in front of you and your toes pointed toward the ceiling. Raise your arms straight out in front of you and pull the tea towel taut.

B. Slowly roll your upper body back, keeping your feet together and continuing to pull the tea towel taut.

C. Continue to roll back until you are lying on your back.

D. From your prone position, slowly roll up until you reach a sitting position with your arms above your head.

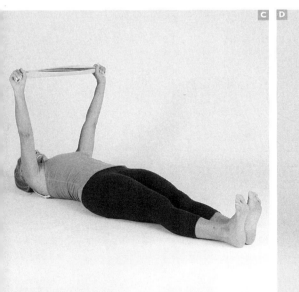
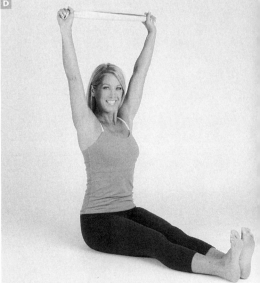

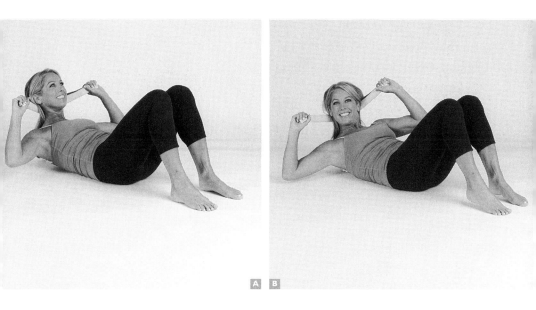

Neck Relaxer Crunch

This is an easy, gentle, natural way to flatten the tummy.

A. Lie on your back. Holding the towel at both ends, place it at the nape of your neck and let it cradle your head and neck almost like a hammock. Bend your knees and place your feet flat on the floor. Now do your crunch: Tighten your abs as you raise your head, neck, and shoulder blades from the floor. Pause, lower, and repeat.

B. For an extra challenge, twist slightly to each side as you raise up, alternating sides.

Double Leg Stretch

This move targets the entire abdominal region—it's a complete ab workout.

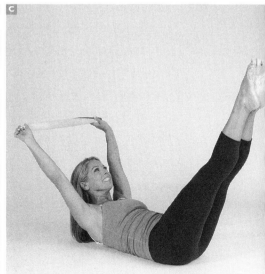

A. Lie on your back, holding the towel taut over your head. Extend your legs up toward the ceiling, with your toes pointed up, and tighten your abs. Exhale as you lift your shoulders slightly off the floor.

B. Keeping your arms extended and the towel taut, bring your knees toward your chest. At the same time, lower your extended arms until the towel is behind your heels.

C. Then, raise your arms over your head, drawing your navel in and keeping the towel taut, and extend your legs. Repeat once more.

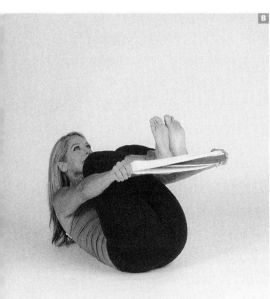

Seat Belt Tap

This exercise focuses on the lower tummy, below the belly button.

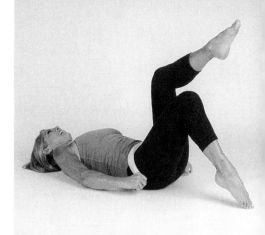

A. Lie on your back. Raise your legs and bend your knees so that they form a ninety-degree angle. Place the towel over your hips to anchor them to the floor and keep your tummy flat. Lower your right leg and tap your right toe to the floor. Return to the starting position, then lower your left leg and tap your left toe to the floor. Alternate toe taps. Try to stabilize your abs as your legs move.

Waistline Trimmer

This trims and slims the oblique muscles—a great rotational exercise for the waistline to cinch in an inch!

A. Come to a sitting position on the floor, with your knees bent. Holding the towel taut, extend your arms straight out in front of you. With toes pointed forward, lift both legs. Twist your upper body first to the left, and then to the right. Continue to twist, alternating sides.

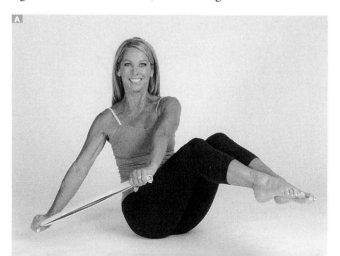

To Calm and Refresh: 5-Minute Balance/Power Moves

Iron Cross

Inspired by my gymnastics days, this move simulates the Iron Cross on the rings to strengthen your arms and shoulders and trim and slim your thighs. You can do it with light weights for extra challenge.

A. Stand tall with your elbows out to the sides and your hands curled into loose fists by your ears. Bend your right knee slightly so just your toes touch the floor.

B. Take a step back with your right foot as you lunge down.

C. Now, using your abs, raise your right knee to waist level as you stand back up.

D. Extend your right leg straight out as you press your arms out to the side, so you form the letter T. (To make the move easier, keep your heel on the floor as you extend your arms.) Repeat for 30 seconds, then switch legs.

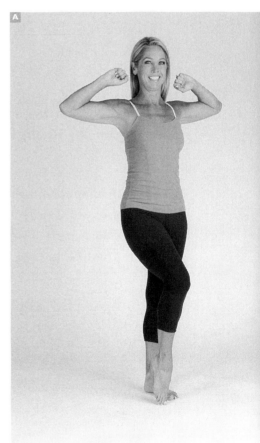

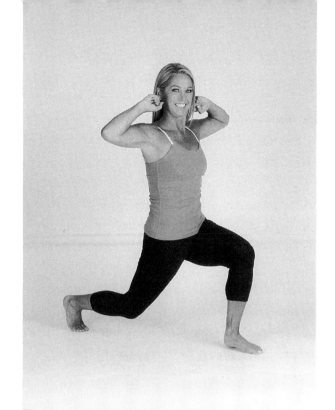

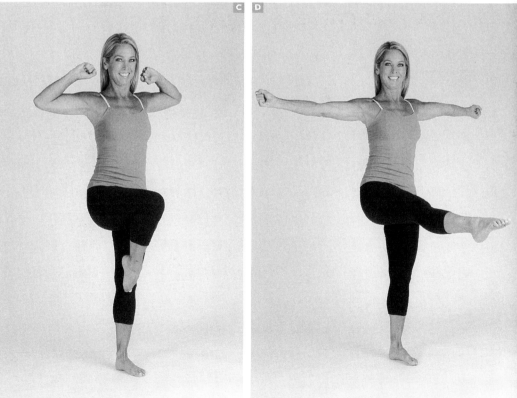

Tightrope Twist

This exercise target-trims your waistline and firms your inner thighs.

A. Stand tall, arms straight out to the sides, with your right foot in front of your left a few inches apart in a straight line, as if you're balancing on a tightrope or on the balance beam.

B. Keep your abs tight and your inner thighs squeezed as you twist to the right for two counts (pulsing), and then back to the center. Make sure your abs are engaged. Repeat for 30 seconds, then switch feet and twist to the left side.

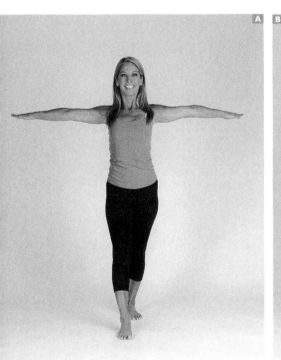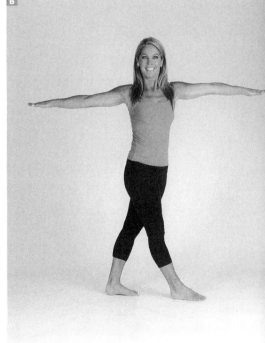

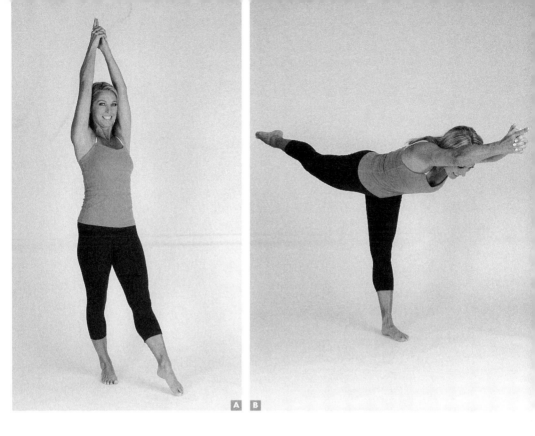

A   B

Balancing Stick

This move is the ultimate total-body toner—it uses every muscle in the body.

A. Stand tall, with your back straight. Raise your arms over your head, interlace your fingers, and point your index fingers toward the ceiling, like temple hands. Bring your left foot forward and touch your toe to the floor.

B. Shift your weight to your left foot and raise your right leg behind you. Hinge your upper body forward from your hips as you slowly continue to raise your right leg. At the same time, keep your abs engaged and bring the rest of your body parallel to the floor. Your body should be one straight line from your pointed index fingers to the big toe of your left foot. Hold for 15 seconds, relax, and repeat on the other side. Repeat once more per side.

Locust

This move strengthens your spine, stretches your arms, and helps prevent carpal tunnel syndrome.

A. Lie on your belly and lift your hips up to place your arms under them, with your palms down, chin resting on the floor. Your ultimate goal is to try to touch your pinkies underneath you. Tighten your abs and buttocks as you raise your right leg, keeping it as straight as you can. Gaze forward, keeping your neck straight and your chin on the floor. Hold for 15 seconds, breathing normally, then relax. Repeat with your other leg. Repeat once more per side. You should feel the stretch in your back, as well as your elbows and forearms.

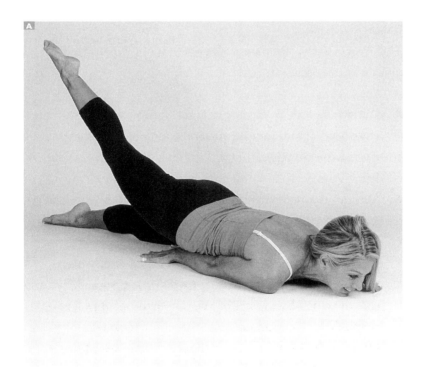

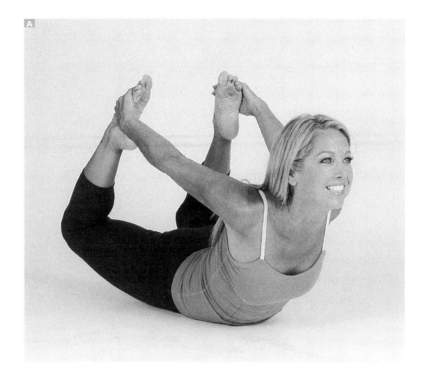

Full Bow

This exercise strengthens your back for natural flexibility of the spine.

A. Lie on your tummy with your arms at your sides. Exhale as you bend your knees until your heels are close to your buttocks. Gently reach back to grasp the outsides of your feet, first the right, then the left, wrapping your fingers two inches from your toes. Make sure your movement is smooth and fluid. With your knees and ankles about eight inches apart, draw your legs up and away from your buttocks, and lift your thighs off the floor. Keeping your head lifted, hold, breathing normally, then relax.

Conclusion

In these pages, I've told you everything I know about how to reclaim your energy so that you can live your life to the fullest. Just as important, I've given you a plan. But never forget that it is you—the beautiful, unique being you are—who must transform this plan from words on a page into action.

Believe that you can rediscover the energy you once had, then act on that belief. Stretch your muscles. Take deep, cleansing breaths. Turn negative feelings into positive action. Nourish your body with good food, and your soul with pleasure. Give yourself permission to sleep and to take time for yourself.

Above all, care for yourself as you care for the people you love. Because when you get right down to it, energy is fueled by a passion for life. Nourish that passion every day, and you will be rewarded in ways you can't yet imagine. You'll be happier, healthier...and unstoppable!

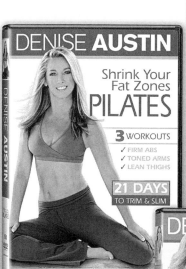
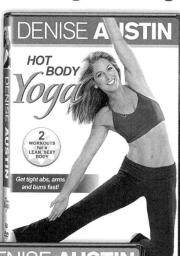
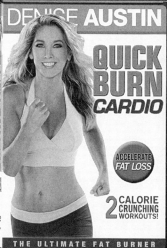 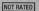

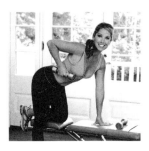